EQUITY, DIVERSITY & INCLUSION
FOR NURSING ASSOCIATES

Sara Miller McCune founded Sage Publishing in 1965 to support the dissemination of usable knowledge and educate a global community. Sage publishes more than 1000 journals and over 800 new books each year, spanning a wide range of subject areas. Our growing selection of library products includes archives, data, case studies and video. Sage remains majority owned by our founder and after her lifetime will become owned by a charitable trust that secures the company's continued independence.

Los Angeles | London | New Delhi | Singapore | Washington DC | Melbourne

EQUITY, DIVERSITY & INCLUSION

FOR NURSING ASSOCIATES

Jacqueline Chang

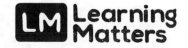

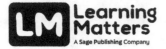

Learning Matters
A Sage Publishing Company
1 Oliver's Yard
55 City Road
London EC1Y 1SP

Sage Publications Inc.
2455 Teller Road
Thousand Oaks, California 91320

Sage Publications India Pvt Ltd
B 1/I 1 Mohan Cooperative Industrial Area
Mathura Road
New Delhi 110 044

Sage Publications Asia-Pacific Pte Ltd
3 Church Street
#10-04 Samsung Hub
Singapore 049483

Editor: Martha Cunneen
Development editors: Sarah Turpie and Ruth Lilly
Senior project editor: Chris Marke
Project managment: Westchester Publishing Services UK
Cover design: Wendy Scott
Marketing manager: Ruslana Khatagova
Typeset by: C&M Digitals (P) Ltd, Chennai, India

Library of Congress Control Number: 2023951111

British Library Cataloguing in Publication Data

A catalogue record for this book is available from the British Library

ISBN 978-1-5296-2299-7
ISBN 978-1-5296-2298-0 (pbk)

Contents

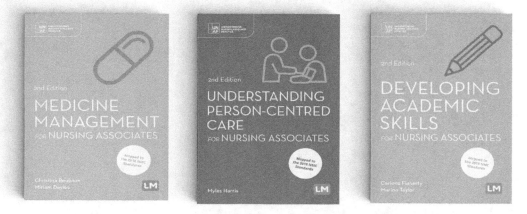

Acknowledgements

Writing this book has been a great personal challenge and I must thank all the support that Sage has given me throughout the whole process.

I would also like to thank my husband Joe and our children Jacob, Thomas and Amy for their patience and support throughout this experience.

And to my parents for always believing.

About the author

Jacqueline Chang qualified as a registered nurse in 2001. She has worked in a variety of settings including cardiac care, oncology, community nursing and palliative care. As well as a BSc in Adult Nursing, Jacqueline has a MA in Medical Ethics and Law which led her into nurse education in 2010. Jacqueline became a Nursing and Midwifery Council recognised teacher in 2012 and has been proud to be involved in teaching and leading nursing associate courses since 2017.

Introduction

Who is this book for?

This book is designed specifically for trainee and qualified nursing associates. However, the content is transferable and relevant for all healthcare professionals. The subject of this book is applicable for everyone working with patients and their families and will provide support for all.

Book structure

Chapter 1: Professional standards

This chapter acts as an overall introduction to the whole book. It will define key terms and look at key legislation and guidelines including the Nursing and Midwifery Council (NMC) Equality, Diversity and Inclusivity (EDI) Plan of 2022, the Standards of Proficiency for Nursing Associates of 2018, the Code of 2018 and the statutory duty of candour of 2014 to identify key professional responsibly for EDI in healthcare. Professional accountability and specifically the role of the nursing associate will be discussed and outlined and related to the importance of being aware of EDI in the nursing associate role. An introduction to key ethical theories will also be given here. This chapter will highlight the importance of EDI in the complex society in which we live and work.

Chapter 2: Legal requirements

The Human Rights Act 1998 and the Equality Act 2010 and the protected characteristics will be outlined and related to healthcare practice. Relevant cases related to discrimination will be used to identify real discrimination issues and abuse in healthcare. These cases will be discussed using the four principles of biomedical ethics (Beauchamp and Childress, 2019) to critically explore the issues raised.

Chapter 3: Exploring unconscious bias

Unconscious bias will be defined and explained with some reflective exercises to help the nursing associate understand their own unconscious bias. The importance of recognising and acknowledging unconscious bias will be discussed, including methods to minimise the impact of unconscious bias. Examples of unconscious bias will be applied to all the protected characteristics of the Human Rights Act to highlight how prevalent unconscious bias is.

Chapter 4: Exploring diversity

The UK is a diverse country, and some geographical areas are more culturally diverse than others. Some differences in various areas of the country will be outlined to demonstrate the challenges for people who may not feel that they are easily accepted by society. Diversity will be defined and social dynamics and social policy in UK healthcare will be introduced in this chapter and explored. Strategies for understanding the social diversity of a particular area in order to identify health inequalities will also be provided in this chapter to help nursing associates understand their own area better.

Chapter 5: Exploring inclusion

The importance of inclusion will be explored in this chapter, including the different access to healthcare in the UK. The changing dynamics of the LGBTQIA+ community will also be explored, linking to current legislation and real-life scenarios impacting on service users. In this chapter we also consider various forms of discrimination and stigmatisation. Cases from UK law will be used to show the growth and development of inclusion in this country, with an indication of how inclusion can be expanded.

Chapter 6: Exploring equity and equality

Equity will be defined and explored, comparing it to equality and looking at the ethical principle of justice. Cases will be used to demonstrate the social injustice in healthcare practice and the impact of this on society with perspectives from both equity and equality. Practical issues will be identified with strategies to enable the nursing associate to manage equity well on a day-to-day basis. An honest exploration of the racism within healthcare will be discussed with ideas for strategies to challenge barriers to care.

Chapter 7: Delivering person-centred care

Person-centred care will be explored with explanations of how to deliver this while considering the requirements of EDI. This will include issues like continued patient assessment and end-of-life care. The specific role of the nursing associate within the multidisciplinary team will be considered. Communication skills will be discussed, including verbal and nonverbal methods of communication. Real-life scenarios will be used to apply the theory to practice and an honest representation of the challenges faced in healthcare practice will be presented.

Chapter 8: Application of EDI to practice

This book will conclude with tips for maintaining EDI principles in practice in UK healthcare. This chapter will act as a summary to the whole book and use key case studies to enable nursing associates to see how to provide unbiased person-centred care at all times.

Requirements for the *NMC Standards of Proficiency for Nursing Associates*

The NMC has established standards of proficiency to be met by applicants to different parts of the register, and these are the standards it considers necessary for safe and effective practice. This book is structured so that it will help you to understand and meet the proficiencies required for entry to the NMC register as a nursing associate. The relevant proficiencies are presented at the start of each chapter so that you can clearly see which ones the chapter addresses. The proficiencies have been designed to be generic so apply to all fields of nursing and all care settings. This is because all nursing associates must be able to meet the needs of any person they encounter in their practice regardless of their stage of life or health challenges, whether these are mental, physical, cognitive or behavioural.

This book includes the latest standards for 2018 onwards, taken from the Standards of Proficiency for Nursing Associates (NMC, 2018b).

Learning features

Textbooks can be intimidating and learning from reading text is not always easy. However, this series has been designed specifically to help the nursing associate learn from the books within it. By using a number of learning features throughout the books, they will help you to develop your understanding and ability to apply theory to practice, while remaining engaging and breaking the text up into manageable chunks. This book contains activities, case studies, theory summary boxes, further reading, useful websites and other materials to enable you to participate in your own learning. The book cannot provide all the answers – but instead provides a good outline of the most important information and helps you build a framework for your own learning.

Professional standards

NMC STANDARDS OF PROFICIENCY FOR NURSING ASSOCIATES

This chapter will address the following platforms and proficiencies:

Platform 1: Being an accountable professional

1.1   understand and act in accordance with the Code: Professional standards of practice and behaviour for nurses, midwives, and nursing associates, and fulfil all registration requirements

1.2   understand and apply relevant legal, regulatory and governance requirements, policies, and ethical frameworks, including any mandatory reporting duties, to all areas of practice

1.3   understand the importance of courage and transparency and apply the duty of candour, recognising and reporting any situations, behaviours or errors that could result in poor care outcomes

1.11   provide, promote, and where appropriate advocate for, non-discriminatory, person-centred and sensitive care at all times. Reflect on people's values and beliefs, diverse backgrounds, cultural characteristics, language requirements, needs and preferences, taking account of any need for adjustments

1.12   recognise and report any factors that may adversely impact safe and effective care provision

1.14   demonstrate the ability to keep complete, clear, accurate and timely records

1.15   take responsibility for continuous self-reflection, seeking and responding to support and feedback to develop professional knowledge and skills

1.16   act as an ambassador for their profession and promote public confidence in health and care services

Platform 5: Improving safety and quality of care

5.6   understand and act in line with local and national organisational frameworks, legislation and regulations to report risks, and implement actions as instructed, following up and escalating as required

5.8   understand when to seek appropriate advice to manage a risk and avoid compromising quality of care and health outcomes

5.9   recognise uncertainty and demonstrate an awareness of strategies to develop resilience in themselves. Know how to seek support to help deal with uncertain situations

5.10   understand their own role and the roles of all other staff at different levels of experience and seniority in the event of a major incident

Chapter aims

After reading this chapter, you will be able to:

- review the role of the nursing associate;
- understand the way that the principles of equity, diversity and inclusivity (EDI) are encompassed in the Code (2018a) and the Standards of Proficiency for Nursing Associates (2018b);
- explore a selection of ethical theories that relate to healthcare;
- identify relevant legislation that informs EDI in healthcare.

Understanding the theory: key terminology

We will begin with a definition of the following key terms, which will be explored throughout the book:

Equality – the principle of providing the same service for everyone. On the surface this seems fair for everybody and a good example of justice.

Equity – the principle of providing specific services for specific people based on personal needs. This is the underlying principle for person-centred care. This has a close link with justice.

Diversity – the understanding that people, among other things, are different. We have a beautifully rich culture with a range of ethnic and cultural backgrounds and these differences need to be embraced and welcomed and learned from.

Inclusivity – recognising the diversity and providing equitable access for everyone to help people who might otherwise not have had access.

Discrimination – treating someone differently due to a feature of theirs, for example race, ethnicity or gender.

Oppression – unjust and unfair treatment.

Introduction

This chapter serves as an introduction to the whole book and defines key terms that will be used throughout. It will introduce important legislation that impacts the day-to-day work of the nursing associate, including the National Health Service (NHS) Constitution, the Code, the Standards of Proficiency, duty of candour and Nursing and Midwifery Council (NMC) frameworks for improving provisions in its practice for EDI. It will also introduce ethical theories that are related to EDI. Accountability and the role of the nursing associate will also be explored.

The role of the nursing associate, the NMC Code and accountability

The NMC is the regulatory body for all healthcare professionals on their register. It was established in 2002 and its Code was implemented immediately. The Code was written for registered nurses and midwives, and it provided a set of rules to abide by. It did not apply to unregistered healthcare professionals (healthcare assistants and midwifery assistants), but only to those who paid their registration fee to the NMC once they had reached the standard of training stipulated by the NMC. These rules regulate the profession with common expected standards to ensure excellent conduct and behaviour and a high standard of care. The Code sets the conduct expected of all nurses, midwives and nursing associates and it has four principles as shown in Table 1.1.

Table 1.1   The Code's four principles

Prioritise people	Preserve safety
Practise effectively	Promote professionalism and trust

The nursing associate role was adopted by the NMC in 2019 following a successful pilot programme. The role of the nursing associate is to support the registered nurses and provide hands-on, high-quality care in all environments to all patients (NMC, 2018b). Nursing associates work in all settings available to them – in patient's homes, in clinics, in general practitioner (GP) surgeries, in triage, in hospitals, in nursing homes and more. As time goes on, the role of the nursing associate is being further developed and understood, and more opportunities are opening up. The generic nature of the course allows nursing associates to work in any of the four fields of nursing – adult, child, mental health and learning difficulties – around the country. The expanding nature of this role means that, in the future, the nursing associate will work in more and more clinical areas. When nursing associates became recognised by the NMC, the Code was updated to include this role (NMC, 2018a). Nursing associates are therefore regulated in the same way and to the same standards as staff nurses and have the same level of accountability, although for different, role-appropriate actions. As a part of this regulatory body, nursing associates need to work within the Code at all times.

Within the four principles of the Code, it clearly states why EDI is so important. For example, point 1.3 states that assumptions must be avoided, and diversity and individual choices must be recognised, and 1.5 instructs all registered healthcare professionals to both respect and uphold the human rights of all. It guides people on the register to prioritise people in need and it also instructs registered professionals to always uphold the reputation of their respective profession. This means being a good role model with high integrity. The expectation of good role modelling is applicable when facing service users and when working with other professionals as well as in day-to-day life.

Everyone registered with the NMC, including all nursing associates, are accountable for their practice. This means that you are answerable to the NMC should you work outside your scope of practice or act in a way which is contradictory to the Code. By being accountable you can be presented to a fitness to practise panel should it be felt that you do not practise in accordance with the Code. Your registration with the NMC can be suspended or you can be removed from the register if your standard of practice is compromised.

The wide application of the nursing associate means that a good understanding and knowledge of EDI is essential for all nursing associates.

NMC Standards for Nursing Associates

The NMC published the Standards for Nursing Associates in 2018 and this consists of six platforms and two annexes. This document outlines exactly what the nursing associate should be able to do once registered with the NMC. The six platforms work through the knowledge and skills that you, as a nursing associate, need to meet in order to register with the NMC. The first platform is titled 'Being an accountable professional' and it clearly outlines the level of accountability that the nursing associate has. Respect and anti-discriminatory behaviour is a key theme within the Standards in order to help protect the service users and the team in which you work.

Proficiency 1.4 expects nursing associates to recognise and report discriminatory behaviour. Proficiency 1.16 asks the nursing associate to act as an ambassador for the profession in order to promote its public image and therefore gain the trust of the public. The only way to do this is to understand the rights of all patients, and then to be courageous enough to act when these rights are ignored. This is what is expected of you as a nursing associate.

Within the platforms and annexes there are direct links made to EDI requirements. These are shown in Table 1.2.

Table 1.2 Platforms and proficiencies linking to EDI (NMC, 2018b)

1.2	understand and apply relevant legal, regulatory and governance requirements, policies, and ethical frameworks, including any mandatory reporting duties, to all areas of practice
1.4	demonstrate an understanding of, and the ability to, challenge or report discriminatory behaviour
1.11	provide, promote, and where appropriate advocate for, nondiscriminatory, person-centred and sensitive care at all times. Reflect on people's values and beliefs, diverse backgrounds, cultural characteristics, language requirements, needs and preferences, taking account of any need for adjustments
2.3	describe the principles of epidemiology, demography, and genomics and how these may influence health and wellbeing outcomes
2.4	understand the factors that may lead to inequalities in health outcomes
3.2	understand and apply the principles and processes for making reasonable adjustments
4.3	understand and apply the principles of human factors and environmental factors when working in teams
6.4	understand the principles and processes involved in supporting people and families with a range of care needs to maintain optimal independence and avoid unnecessary interventions and disruptions to their lives
6.5	identify when people need help to facilitate equitable access to care, support and escalate concerns appropriately
Annex A	It will be important for nursing associates to demonstrate cultural awareness when caring for people and to ensure that the needs, priorities, expertise and preferences of people are always valued and taken into account.
Annex A	Where people have special communication needs or a disability, it is essential that nursing associates make reasonable adjustments. This means they'll be able to provide and share information in a way that promotes good health and health outcomes and does not prevent people from having equal access to the highest quality of care

Once you have explored the professional rules and regulations that support nursing associates, we will consider the ethical theories that help to support decision-making in healthcare.

Principles of biomedical ethics

The principles of biomedical ethics were first outlined in 1977 (see Beauchamp and Childress, 2019) and are still relevant today. They will always be relevant. There are four principles in this ethical theory: autonomy, beneficence, justice and non-maleficence. There is some debate as to which principle is the most important and Gillon (2003) argues that autonomy is the most important, while others argue that non-maleficence should be a priority principle as to do no harm is central to healthcare. Another opinion is that the priority order of the principles is dependent on the particular situation. Here they are described in alphabetical order to briefly state how they link to EDI.

Autonomy

The principle of autonomy is essential in healthcare as it allows people to make their own decisions about their own healthcare without coercion or an expectation of compliance. Autonomy is about respecting the person in front of us and understanding their personal needs and desires regarding their own health. To do this we need to know what is important to them and understand their personal requirements. This is the essence of person-centred care, and all nursing associates must work promoting person-centred care. In order to promote autonomy, the nursing associate needs to take the time to listen to their patient and find out what their preferences are.

Consent to treatment is only valid if the patient is allowed to make decisions for themselves once all the information has been given to them. This is intrinsically linked to autonomy. The decision must be made by the patient but if they want to discuss this with a family member then that would be fine, as long as the decision is theirs. If the person is unable to give consent, then family members are well placed to advise what the person would have wanted. This can help to promote autonomy for the patient even if they cannot make decisions themselves.

Once a person reaches the age of 18, they provide their own consent unless they lack the capacity to do so. If there is a lasting power of attorney (LPA) for health in place, then that LPA can make decisions where necessary. If there is no LPA, then, when decisions are made on behalf of a patient, it is expected that all decisions made are in the best interests of the patient and that the decision made is as close to the decision that the patient would have made themselves were they able to (Mental Capacity Act 2005).

Beneficence

The principle of beneficence is thought of as being kind and caring to the service users and patients. However, it is much more than that. It is not only working in the best interests of the person in your care, but it is also doing the best you can for them. By understanding the person in front of you, you are able to provide the care that they want. In order to work towards beneficence, the nursing associate needs to understand what that person wants and to understand why they want it. If the person cannot tell you what they want themselves, then it may be appropriate to ask their family what they think the person would want in order to promote beneficence as much as possible. In some situations, it may be possible to do the least invasive procedures required until the person is able to communicate and state their choices regarding further treatment.

It is important to remember that beneficence and autonomy are linked. What is in the patient's best interests may be a matter of opinion. What the patient wants and what the healthcare professionals think they should have are not always the same and the voice of the patient must be heard. It is also important to remember that extending life is not always in the best interests of the patient. Stopping treatment and allowing someone to have the best death they can may be in the person's best interests and that can be difficult to accept sometimes. End-of-life care will be explored further in Chapter 7.

Justice

When thinking about EDI, the ethical principle of justice is clearly linked. The NHS Constitution (GOV.UK, 2023a) has seven principles and the first one is the principle that the service it provides is available to every person who needs it. It states clearly that human rights will be respected and that social inequalities will be assessed and focused on. Justice, as an ethical principle, looks at the fairness of treatment allocated to each individual. All nursing associates have a responsibility to be fair when caring for their patients and their patient's families. Fairness applies to many different elements of healthcare. On a large scale, fairness is a strategic consideration when allocating NHS funds to services. On an everyday scale, when you decide how much time to give to each patient that you are looking after, you are working using the principle of justice. It is distributive justice. Allocation of care is a part of justice that is seen every day and there are different ways in which you can allocate yourself and these all have an impact on patients and their families. Activity 1.1 asks you to consider different ways in which care can be distributed.

Activity 1.1   Critical thinking

Consider the following list of principles of distributive justice provided by Beauchamp and Childress (2019):

- To each person an equal share.
- To each person according to need.
- To each person according to effort.
- To each person according to contribution.
- To each person according to merit.
- To each person according to free-market exchanges.

Which do you think is the most important one to you and why?

Have you ever had patients or families challenge you regarding how you distributed your care?
  An outline answer is provided at the end of the chapter.

Non-maleficence

This is the principle of not doing any harm to your patients. It should be noted, however, that neglecting to prevent harm is just as destructive as intentionally causing harm. Being a patient's advocate is an essential element of the nursing associate's role. Understanding the diversity of people and ensuring that others also respect this diversity is part of healthcare delivery.

Harm is caused to your patients regularly and ideally these are expected harms. For example, giving someone a medication for their pain knowing that this medication will cause them to feel nauseated is an expected harm caused by your action. Another example is performing venepuncture and causing a bruise. It doesn't always happen, but it is a known and expected harm that is common in healthcare. These harms are acknowledged and expected by the doctrine of double effect (Brueck and Sulmasy, 2020). The doctrine has four conditions (Salmasy, 2007):

- The action itself is good or at least neutral.
- The good effect, not the bad effect, is what is intended.
- The good effect is not produced by the bad effect.
- There is a proportionately grave reason for permitting the bad effect.

Although it is hoped, and to an extent, assumed, that healthcare professionals will always endeavour to not intentionally cause harm, and as long as the action made meets the criteria of the doctrine of double effect, then there is no issue. Some harms are expected, acknowledged and accepted as part of healthcare. The importance here is knowing the intention of the action in the first place. As a nursing associate you must ensure that all your actions are necessary for the treatment of the person in front of you. As well as delivering your own care, you act as an advocate for your patient, ensuring all care delivered is required and minimal harm is caused by any member of the multidisciplinary team (NMC, 2018b).

As stated, the four principles are not given an order of priority; all are as important as each other. However, in reality you may feel that you focus on one more than the others, depending on the situation that you are in.

Activity 1.2   Reflection

Thinking about the four principles – autonomy, beneficence, justice and non-maleficence – which one do you think you put the most emphasis on in your day-to-day work?

Is there a principle that you don't consider on a day-to-day basis?
An outline answer is provided at the end of the chapter.

The principles of biomedical ethics is a well-used theory in healthcare and will always be relevant in healthcare. However, there are other ethical theories that also have their place in healthcare. Two further theories are described here:

- Consequentialism is the theory that the best thing to do is what causes the most benefit for the greatest number of people (Sinnott-Armstrong, 2022).
- Deontology is the theory that people must always do what is right, even if the outcomes are not as desirable as you might like (Alexander and Moore, 2021). It is the duty of doing the right thing that is important in deontology.

Ethical theories are useful when decisions need to be made. Decisions are made on many different levels – strategic, local and personal – and you will make decisions every day at work, for example, when you decide in what order to help patients with their hygiene needs, or when you decide when to allocate an appointment to someone. All of these everyday decisions require some ethical decision-making regarding the needs of the patient and the availability of services, although you may not consciously consider ethical theories at the time.

The following two case studies ask you to consider everyday issues and make your decision using ethical theories to support you.

Case study: Medication round

You are working in an adult surgical ward. You are working in a bay of six patients and two side rooms, and you have a Band 2 working with you while the Band 5 nurse is overseeing the ward and administering intravenous medication. You have completed the morning oral medication administration for your patients and worked with the Band 2 to assist with personal hygiene needs. It is now lunchtime and two patients have rung their bell and are asking for help to go to the toilet. As it is lunchtime the ward is low on numbers due to staff breaks, and the staff nurse is administering the lunchtime intravenous medications around the ward. You have started the lunchtime medication round.

Activity 1.3   Decision-making

How do you decide what to do when and why?

- Do you call for further help and continue with the medication round?
- Do you stop the medication round and help the patients go to the toilet?
- How do you decide which patient to take to the toilet first?

How can you justify your decision using ethical theories?
An outline answer is provided at the end of the chapter.

Case study: GP surgery

You are working in a GP surgery and your next appointment is for venepuncture on a patient you do not know. The patient comes in and sits down and you notice that he is anxious and appears to be distressed. You ask him how he is and he starts to cry. He opens up to you and tells you that he has been struggling recently with finding work and he is worried about supporting his family. He feels that he does not know what to do and states that his life is not worth living any more and that his family will be better off without him. He suddenly stands up to leave and it is clear he is going to get into his car. You're concerned that he will try to end his life using his car.

Activity 1.4   Decision-making

After reading the above case study, consider the following:

- What can you do?
- Should you call the police and stop him? What will this mean for him?
- What is your role here as a nursing associate?

Justify your decision-making process using consequentialism and deontology.
An outline answer is provided at the end of the chapter.

The NHS Constitution

The NHS has been a feature of the United Kingdom since 1947. It is a phenomenal, unique health service that a lot of people take for granted at times. The NHS has a constitution which is made up of seven principles and six values. They are outlined in Tables 1.3 and 1.4.

Table 1.3   The seven principles of the NHS Constitution (GOV.UK, 2023a)

1	The NHS provides a comprehensive service, available to all	The NHS is available to all irrespective of gender, race, disability, age, sexual orientation, religion, belief, gender reassignment, pregnancy, and maternity or marital or civil partnership status. The service is designed to improve, prevent, diagnose, and treat both physical and mental health problems with equal regard. It has a duty to each and every individual that it serves and must respect their human rights. At the same time, it has a wider social duty to promote equality through the services it provides and to pay particular attention to groups or sections of society where improvements in health and life expectancy are not keeping pace with the rest of the population.
2	Access to NHS services is based on clinical need, not an individual's ability to pay	NHS services are free of charge, except in limited circumstances sanctioned by Parliament.
3	The NHS aspires to the highest standards of excellence and professionalism	It provides high-quality care that is safe, effective, and focused on patient experience; in the people it employs, and in the support, education, training, and development they receive; in the leadership and management of its organisations; and through its commitment to innovation and to the promotion, conduct and use of research to improve the current and future health and care of the population. Respect, dignity, compassion, and care should be at the core of how patients and staff are treated not only because that is the right thing to do but because patient safety, experience and outcomes are all improved when staff are valued, empowered, and supported.
4	The patient will be at the heart of everything the NHS does	The NHS should support individuals to promote and manage their own health. NHS services must reflect, and should be coordinated around and tailored to, the needs and preferences of patients, their families, and their carers. As part of this, the NHS will ensure that in line with the Armed Forces Covenant, those in the armed forces, reservists, their families, and veterans are not disadvantaged in accessing health services in the area they reside. Patients, with their families and carers, where appropriate, will be involved in and consulted on all decisions about their care and treatment. The NHS will actively encourage feedback from the public, patients, and staff, welcome it and use it to improve its services.

(Continued)

Table 1.3   (Continued)

5	The NHS works across organisational boundaries	The NHS works in partnership with other organisations in the interest of patients, local communities, and the wider population. The NHS is an integrated system of organisations and services bound together by the principles and values reflected in the Constitution. The NHS is committed to working jointly with other local authority services, other public sector organisations and a wide range of private and voluntary sector organisations to provide and deliver improvements in health and wellbeing.
6	The NHS is committed to providing best value for taxpayers' money	The NHS is committed to providing the most effective, fair, and sustainable use of finite resources. Public funds for healthcare will be devoted solely to the benefit of the people that the NHS serves.
7	The NHS is accountable to the public, communities, and patients that it serves	The NHS is a national service funded through national taxation, and it is the government which sets the framework for the NHS, and which is accountable to Parliament for its operation. However, most decisions in the NHS, especially those about the treatment of individuals and the detailed organisation of services, are rightly taken by the local NHS and by patients with their clinicians. The system of responsibility and accountability for taking decisions in the NHS should be transparent and clear to the public, patients, and staff. The government will ensure that there is always a clear and up-to-date statement of NHS accountability for this purpose.

Table 1.4   The six values of the NHS Constitution (GOV.UK, 2023a)

1	Working together for patients	Patients come first in everything we do. We fully involve patients, staff, families, carers, communities, and professionals inside and outside the NHS. We put the needs of patients and communities before organisational boundaries. We speak up when things go wrong.
2	Respect and dignity	We value every person – whether a patient, their families or carers, or staff – as an individual, respect their aspirations and commitments in life, and seek to understand their priorities, needs, abilities, and limits. We take what others have to say seriously. We are honest and open about our point of view and about what we can and cannot do.
3	Commitment to quality of care	We earn the trust placed in us by insisting on quality and striving to get the basics of quality of care – safety, effectiveness, and patient experience – right every time. We encourage and welcome feedback from patients, families, carers, staff, and the public. We use this to improve the care we provide and build on our successes.
4	Compassion	We ensure that compassion is central to the care we provide and respond with humanity and kindness to each person's pain, distress, anxiety or need. We search for the things we can do, however small, to give comfort and relieve suffering. We find time for patients, their families, and carers, as well as those we work alongside. We do not wait to be asked, because we care.

| 5 | Improving lives | We strive to improve health and wellbeing and people's experiences of the NHS. We cherish excellence and professionalism wherever we find it – in the everyday things that make people's lives better as much as in clinical practice, service improvements and innovation. We recognise that all have a part to play in making ourselves, patients, and our communities healthier. |
| 6 | Everyone counts | We maximise our resources for the benefit of the whole community, and make sure nobody is excluded, discriminated against, or left behind. We accept that some people need more help, that difficult decisions must be taken – and that when we waste resources, we waste opportunities for others. |

The NMC EDI Plan

In 2022, NHS Digital revealed that approximately 1.3 million people work for the NHS and, according to the registration data from the NMC, of these 1.3 million employees, approximately 771,000 are registered with the NMC.

The workforce data collected by the NHS in 2022 is shown in Figure 1.1.

| 68% are women | 37% identify as BAME | 8% have a disability | 5.5% are lesbian, gay | 49.2% have a religion | 53.2% are under 39 |

Figure 1.1 NHS workforce data (NHS Digital, 2022)

As must be expected, not all of the employees of the NHS completed and returned the surveys, so there is an acknowledgement that the data cannot be assumed to be 100 per cent accurate. However, companies can only work with the data they are given, which is what the NMC is doing. What the figures do show is a diverse community in one very big organisation. This diversity indicates the need for understanding, acceptance and equity within the organisation. Unfortunately, within the NHS there are reports of racism and unfairness. For example, research conducted by the NMC in 2022 found that the greatest number of fitness to practise referrals were for Black professionals and for male employees (NMC, 2022c). These two groups have a strong feeling of unfair treatment and a lack of equity in their employment as they feel that there are double standards within their workplace. Their complaint is not unfounded, as each region of the NHS has a statement and plan to tackle racism. Some make mention of other groups that are discriminated against, but the focus, for most, is that of racism. It is important to see that institutional racism within the NHS is being identified across the country. It is also important to understand that the prejudice comes from not only service users but from staff members as well, and it also appears in promotion decisions and in recognition of achievement.

Activity 1.5   Reflection

Consider your own ethnic background:

- Do you feel that you are treated the same as everyone else in your workplace?
- Have you ever seen anyone treated differently which may have been due to their ethnicity?

(Continued)

(Continued)

- What does the senior management in your place of work look like?
- Is it multicultural, or is there a high number of a certain group?
- Does this reflect the geographical area in which you work?

As this is a personal reflection, no outline answer is provided at the end of the chapter.

The NMC hopes to reduce the occurrence of this discrimination with their 2022 plan. The NMC published their EDI Plan (NMC, 2022c), which is to be implemented between 2022 and 2025. The intention of this plan is to provide a safe working environment for everyone on the register. It sets out an action plan to allow everyone to be able to work without fearing bias and discrimination. This plan forms part of the NMC Corporate Plan for 2022–2025 (NMC, 2022b) to support the goal of making the NMC processes fair for all employees. The plan is focused on staff only as the NMC wants to increase inclusivity for all employees, which will in turn increase the confidence that our service users have in the system.

The NMC EDI Plan (NMC, 2022c) has four objectives which are shown in Table 1.5.

Table 1.5 The NMC EDI Plan objectives

A	Reflect our values as a regulator that prioritises the needs and wellbeing of the nursing and midwifery professional and the public.
B	Make sure we show good equality practice as an employer.
C	Use EDI data in a strategic and coordinated way, both internally and with partners across the health and care sector.
D	Tackle health inequalities by using our platform to advocate for better care for everyone accessing services.

The NMC has ten priority themes in this plan, as shown in Table 1.6.

Table 1.6 Priority themes from the NMC Corporate Plan (2022b)

1	Take a more sophisticated approach to collecting and using EDI data.
2	Learn from EDI evidence to create targeted interventions.
3	Co-produce EDI solutions through collaboration with informed, diverse external partners.
4	Enhance the EDI competency and accountability of our leaders.
5	Enhance the EDI capability of all colleagues.
6	Map and improve EDI-informed decision-making.
7	Address evidence of discrimination or barriers in our processes.
8	Use our influence to support the prevention and reduction of health inequalities.
9	Strengthen our EDI governance.
10	Use regulatory reform as a vehicle to embed EDI in our structures and ways of working.

While this is a three-year plan, the NMC makes it clear that a new plan will be written for 2025 onwards as supporting staff in an ever-changing world is not a task that will ever be completed. It will need to be re-worked and re-written constantly. Complacency is not an option when working with EDI needs as the community in which we live and work is constantly changing.

As a patient-facing professional, you, as a nursing associate, need to be constantly reflecting, updating and developing yourself.

This chapter will now explore the Parliamentary Acts that protect vulnerable people in the UK.

The Human Rights Act 1998

The Human Rights Act was developed in 1998 and became legal in the UK in 2000. The Act took specific points from the European Convention of Human Rights (ECHR) (Council of Europe, 1950) and made them UK law. There are 14 articles in the Act and 4 protocols, as opposed to 59 articles and 16 protocols in the ECHR. The intention was to protect citizens of the UK and ensure fair and equitable treatment for all.

The Human Rights Act applies to everyone in the UK from birth to death and they are applicable to all with no prejudice. They cannot be removed, although they can be restricted to protect public safety. All these rights are essential to living in today's society, but some relate particularly to EDI and these are the ones highlighted in Table 1.7.

Table 1.7 The Human Rights Act articles relating to EDI

Article 8	states that everyone has a 'right to respect your private life, your family life, your home and your correspondence'.
Article 9	protects the right to 'freedom of thought, conscience and religion'.
Article 10	protects the 'freedom of expression'.
Article 12	protects the 'right to marry' for 'men and women of marriageable age'.
Article 14	protects people from discrimination based on protected characteristics from the Equality Act (2010).

The Equality Act 2010

The Equality Act was introduced as an addition to the Human Rights Act to legally protect people from discrimination in all parts of society. Through research and investigation, it was found that employers would make an effort to not employ certain people and if they were employed, they would get a lower salary than other employees of equal experience doing the same job. To discriminate against someone in this way has an impact on their ability to access healthcare, which has implications for the health of the nation. It is not uncommon for people to be discriminated against and the Equality Act protects nine specific characteristics from discrimination, which are shown in Figure 1.2.

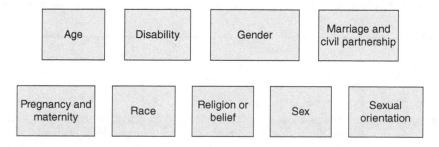

Figure 1.2 Protected characteristics under the Equality Act 2010

The characteristics were identified as a means to challenge the inequalities in health and funding that people in these groups are subjected to. It demands that people are given a fair chance to employment, to education and to pay, and that decisions are not made to disadvantage people because of a protected characteristic. The protected characteristics reassure all members of society that decisions about employment, housing, education, access to health services and joining any clubs will not be made based on prejudice against one of the nine characteristics. They apply to all members of society, and all hate crimes based on any of these characteristics are illegal. As a nursing associate you are expected to treat everyone to the best of your ability and not treat anyone differently based on a protected characteristic. The Equality Act will be looked at in more detail in Chapter 6.

Duty of candour

In 2015 the NMC published their duty of candour guidance in coalition with the General Medical Council; it has subsequently been updated over the last few years (NMC, 2022a). The duty of candour guides those registered with the NMC to be honest and truthful when things go wrong with a patient's treatment or care and anything that could harm a patient. It is easy to assume that this is reserved for medical treatment, for example, surgery on the wrong part of the body, an arm bruised from venepuncture, or a drug administration error. However, poor care being given because a healthcare professional is not treating the person fairly is still poor care. It is still an error in the care being delivered as no one should be mistreated. Psychological damage caused by prejudicial treatment destroys relationships with the NHS as trust is lost. The impact that this has on the patient and their families is significant. Therefore, the NHS Constitution supports the duty of candour with the following pledge, illustrating how important it is:

> The NHS pledges to ensure that when mistakes happen or if you are harmed while receiving healthcare you receive an appropriate explanation and apology, delivered with sensitivity and recognition of the trauma you have experienced, and know that lessons will be learned to help avoid a similar incident occurring again (GOV.UK, 2023a).

As a nursing associate, if you see improper medical treatment, it is expected that you will escalate your concerns. The expectation is the same if you witness unfair treatment based on race or age, or anything of the protected characteristics. Proficiency 1.3 of the Standards of Proficiency expects all nursing associates to *understand the importance of courage and transparency and apply the duty of candour, recognising and reporting any situations, behaviours or errors that could result in poor care outcomes* (NMC, 2018b), clarifying how important candour is for nursing associates.

To whistleblow against a member of staff is a challenging thing to do. People raising concerns and complaints often worry about harassment or victimisation (NHS England, 2023a) but to protect patients and ensure you are working within the boundaries of the Code with respect to candour it is imperative that all poor care is recognised quickly and reported appropriately.

Chapter summary

The importance of the role of the nursing associate is clear – you need to understand the professional requirements that that are needed when you have people in your care. You have duties under the Human Rights Act and the Equality Act and also from your own personal ethical code. You need to make sure that you work within your scope of practice to uphold the profession that you have chosen to enter. If you do not do this then you could be removed from the NMC register. As a nursing associate you need to recognise potential risks to high-quality patient care, and you need to escalate all concerns appropriately. Your role is patient facing and you are perfectly placed to build relationships with patients and promote their wellbeing in a person-centred manner.

Activities: Brief outline answers

Activity 1.1

It would be nice to be able to give everyone the same care, but the principle of person-centred care does not allow for this. Different people need different levels of care at different times. As a rule, nursing associates will allocate according to need. This may upset some people and you may hear some patients or families complain that they are being neglected when they are not. You might hear people stating that they pay their taxes, or that they fought in the war, or another reason, but as a nursing associate you must prioritise your care based on nursing grounds as that is how you deliver fair and equitable person-centred care.

Activity 1.2

Each principle of biomedical ethics is important, and the priority of the principles will change depending on the situation you are in. On a day-to-day basis it is common to think that we mainly promote autonomy where possible. However, you are always working to do what is best for that patient and you are always trying to cause minimal harm. You also deal with healthcare provision as you yourself are a resource and you allocate yourself accordingly. So, on a day-to-day basis you are constantly using all four principles to guide your actions when you are planning and delivering care. No one principle is more important than any of the others.

Activity 1.3

You need to decide what the highest priority is. Consider the medications that are due and whether any are to be administered at a specific time. You need to think about how to manage this as this would be a priority.

The needs of the patients must come first and, putting yourself in the situation the patients are in, needing to go to the toilet is a priority from their perspective. When deciding which patient needs to go first then you may need to look at whether one could be mobilised on to a commode at the bedside if the other one can then walk to the toilet, if that makes it easier to manage.

It is fine to ask for help from other members of the team as there is only so much you can do on your own, but you need to consider what you are delegating and why. Delegating personal needs to others may not be the best use of the staff who come to help you and you need to consider everyone's scope of practice. It may be best to lock the medication trolley up and deliver the essential care that the patients require at that time.

Activity 1.4

Consequentialism – the consequences of stopping him leaving can be positive or negative. Stopping him may include calling the police, which could have a negative outcome. It would involve undermining his confidence and breaking any trust that had been established. This could have a long-term negative impact on this patient when dealing with healthcare professionals in the future. The consequences of not telling the police are that he could harm himself and others and you might have been able to prevent this. This could be considered negligent on your part.

Deontology – it is your duty to protect your patients and the general public. If the patient is posing a risk to himself and others, then you are duty bound to stop him. The theory of deontology considers that the potentially negative outcomes of this are not as important as doing the right thing.

As a nursing associate you are obliged to escalate concerns to appropriate people in accordance with the Code (NMC, 2018a) and you need to explain to the patient that in order to help him you need to share his situation with appropriate members of the team.

Further reading

Council of Europe (1950) European Convention on Human Rights. Available at: **www.echr.coe.int/documents/d/echr/convention_eng**

The full European Convention of Human Rights document.

Useful websites

www.libertyhumanrights.org.uk

For more information on the Human Rights Act.

www.nmc.org.uk

For more information working for the NMC.

Chapter 2

Legal requirements

Chapter aims

After reading this chapter, you will be able to:

- understand the process for making UK laws;
- explore the UK laws that relate to the role of the nursing associate in practice;
- apply relevant UK laws to case studies to support decision-making;
- discuss cases of abuse in healthcare and the role of the nursing associate to promote effective, safe practice.

Introduction

This chapter considers some of the laws and Acts in the UK that relate directly to EDI. It considers various laws and how they relate to healthcare ethics and to the nursing associate, and uses both fictitious and real case scenarios to show the way that ethics and law can work together to promote a high standard of healthcare. It also uses real-life cases to illustrate where substandard care is delivered and explores how the laws and ethics that guide healthcare were ignored in those cases.

Activity 2.1   Evidence-based practice and research

Which of the following statements are true according to UK law?

- It is a legal requirement that you help to save a drowning child.
- It is against the law to park on double red lines.
- It is against the law to kill a swan.
- It is a legal requirement that you must always try to prevent someone from committing suicide.
- It is against the law to drink alcohol and drive a car.
- It is against the law to smoke in a car with a child present.

An outline answer is provided at the end of the chapter.

How law is made in the UK

In the UK, laws are made in Parliament. The UK Parliament has three elements: the House of Commons, the House of Lords and the Head of State (currently King Charles III). The process of making a law is long and has various stages (GOV.UK, 2023b). All three elements of Parliament have to agree to the proposed law for it to actually become law. The new law proposal can come from either the House of Lords or the House of Commons. The process is the same regardless of which house it comes from. We will now examine this process in more detail, looking at each step in turn.

The first step is that someone has an idea for a new law and this proposal is called a 'bill'. That bill can come from either the government itself or from an individual MP. Once the people involved are happy to present that bill, a series of stages occur, as shown in Figure 2.1.

This process can take many years and can be stopped at any point in the process. The bill has to be agreed by both Houses so many law proposals do not get passed and do not become law. More information can be found on this on the UK Parliament website, which can be found in the further reading section at the end of this chapter.

Acts of Parliament

There are some Acts of Parliament which link directly with your day-to-day work as a nursing associate. They include the Human Rights Act of 1998 and the Equality Act of 2010, which we

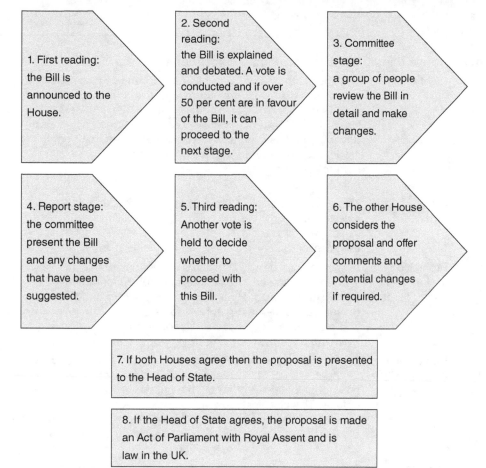

Figure 2.1 A flow chart illustrating the passage of a bill through Parliament to become law

will now examine in more detail. These Acts will be visited in multiple chapters of this book as they need to be considered regularly when advocating and protecting patients in your role as a nursing associate.

The Human Rights Act 1998

The Human Rights Act came into law in the year 2000 and it gives everybody in the UK the right to be treated with dignity, fairness, respect and equality. It was based on the European Convention of Human Rights of 1950. By having a UK-specific Act, citizens of the UK have better access to justice without needing to go to the European Court of Justice.

There are many articles and protocols within the Act which provide protection to all UK citizens and ensure that any new laws are compatible with these rights. The articles that directly relate to healthcare and to EDI are shown in Table 2.1.

Table 2.1   The Human Rights Act 1998

Article number	Article title	What this protects	Exceptions
2	Right to life.	This means that no one has the right to end your life, including the government. It is made clear that the right to life is not a right to death.	A public official can use necessary force to stop a riot, to stop someone committing violence, to make a lawful arrest and to stop someone escaping arrest, and if death is caused during this then that right to life has not been breached.
3	Prohibition of torture.	This article protects everyone from inhumane or degrading treatment or torture.	None. This is an absolute rule.
4	Prohibition of slavery and forced labour.	No person can be 'owned' by another person or be forced to work for someone and are unable to leave the premises.	There are exceptions to this article, for example, compulsory community service, jury duty or exceptional circumstances like natural disasters where the government requires people to help.
5	Right to liberty and security.	This is focused on the right to a fair trial and not be detained unfairly. This also links with the Deprivation of Liberty Safeguards.	People can be detained for the following reasons: fulfilling a prison sentence or awaiting a prison sentence; sectioned under the Mental Health Act; at risk of spreading an infectious disease; is an undocumented immigrant or awaiting deportation or extradition.
8	Right to respect for private and family life.	A right to live privately without government interference. This includes the right to enjoy your family and to enjoy the home in which you live.	Public authorities can restrict your privacy in a proportionate way if there is a risk to national security, public safety or the economy. Other situations include a need to protect health, morals and the rights and freedom of other people and to prevent crimes or public disorders.
9	Freedom of thought, belief and religion.	The right to choose and change your religion and practise your religion.	A person can be prevented from demonstrating their beliefs, thoughts and religion if there is a risk to public safety or order or if people need to be protected from the religious beliefs and actions of another person.
10	Freedom of expression.	The right to express your views.	A public authority may prevent someone from expressing themselves in order to protect national security, territorial integrity or public safety. Or in order to prevent disorder or crime, to protect health and morals and the rights of other people and their reputations and also to prevent any breaches of confidentiality.
14	Prohibition of discrimination.	This makes it illegal to discriminate against people. This is further developed in the Equality Act of 2010.	None. This is absolute.

As a nursing associate it is important to be aware of these Human Rights Act articles because they have an impact on your day-to-day work. Every patient is a vulnerable person and they have a right to be protected under the Act.

The Equality Act 2010

The Equality Act is discussed frequently in this book as it has particular relevance to many different chapters. Within the Equality Act are the nine protected characteristics which are listed and discussed in all of the chapters in this book. As well as the protected characteristics, the Equality Act defines what counts as discrimination and is therefore against the law. It states the duty for adjustments to be made to support people with a disability. It outlines the duties of employers and employees plus pension provision for all. It also clarifies the right to education for all at all levels. It is a detailed Act of over 116 separate legislative pieces, providing protection for anyone with an issue arising from the nine protected characteristics. It is essential that people have an understanding of this Act as it affects every person every day. As a nursing associate you are duty-bound to treat all people equally and fairly without prejudice. This relates to patients, relatives and colleagues.

The Bolam effect

As well as Parliamentary Acts, healthcare legislation is affected by cases that are taken to court. The outcome of a medical law case shows precedent for certain rulings that can then be used in future cases. The following case ruling is applied to medical practice daily.

In 1957, in a case called *Bolam* v *Friern Hospital* (1957), a patient sued his doctor for negligence. He was having electroconvulsive therapy (ECT) and was not given a muscle relaxant, was not restrained, and was not warned of the risks of the treatment procedure. He sustained multiple fractures during the ECT procedure. He therefore had a case for negligence. However, he did not win his case as it was decided that the doctor acted in a reasonable way in accordance with other doctors at that time. At the time of his treatment, people were not always restrained for ECT, and they were not always given a muscle relaxant. Also, in the 1950s people were not told all the risks of their procedures, only the ones the doctors deemed relevant. Three subsequent cases provided further guidance to the Bolam test. In 1997 the ruling in a case dictated that if a medical opinion on diagnosis and treatment is not logical then it can be wrong even if other professionals agree with it (*Bolitho* v *Hackney HA*). In 2004 the case of *Chester* v *Afshar* stated that it is the duty of the doctor to warn the patient of the risks of surgery prior to being asked to consent. In 2015 the judgment in *Montgomery* v *Lanarkshire Health Board* clarified that patients need to be given all the information about their procedures in order to properly consent to them (Lee, 2017). The responsibility of applying the Bolam test, with the subsequent clarifications, lies with the medical professional. When it first came to be used in practice the focus was on its application by doctors only, but as healthcare has evolved, and nurses and nursing associates have become more autonomous, this test now applies to all. All healthcare professionals need to show that they acted in accordance with a body of their peers and their actions were reasonable and appropriate. If they do not pass the Bolam test, then they can be found guilty of negligence and malpractice.

As well as legal limitations, nursing associates are also bound by professional standards from the Code (NMC, 2018a) and the Standards (NMC, 2018b). Within these documents a range of statements are made regarding the role of the nursing associate, including accountability, working within their scope of practice and the support that they will be given.

Accountability

'Accountability' is a word that is important in the Code (NMC, 2018a) and the Standards (NMC, 2018b) as nursing associates are accountable for their practice. This means that all nursing associates need to be able to justify all the decisions that they make and all of the actions that they do, or do not do. All nursing associates may need to explain their actions to others and, potentially, in a law court. As a nursing associate you are accountable, or answerable for, everything that you do. In order to do that you need to understand everything that you are doing, why you are doing it and the implications of doing it. You also always need to be working within your scope of practice and this is made clear in the Standards (NMC, 2018b).

Scope of practice

The Code (2018a) and Standards (2018b) clearly state what is expected of the nursing associate. As a nursing associate you know exactly what you are allowed to do in practice thanks to the Standards. The confusing element of your role is that each NHS Trust, and each clinical area within each Trust, can have specific differences depending on what they need. Some clinical areas will want you to cannulate, for example, while others will not permit you to perform that skill. This means it is essential that you understand your local policies to make sure you are working within your scope of practice. You also need to be competent with any skill you are asked to perform, and if you are not, you need to be open and honest about these development areas.

Vicarious liability

As an employee, your employer has a duty to provide legal protection for you and for the duties that you perform. They are responsible for your actions and omissions at your workplace and therefore provide a level of insurance for you. This is called vicarious liability. There are times, however, when an employer will not support you legally. If you knowingly act outside of your scope of practice and cause harm to a patient, then your employer may decide that they will not support you (NMC, 2022d).

Neglect versus abuse

Neglect and abuse are two words that are used when vulnerable people have suffered at the hands of healthcare professionals. They have different meanings and implications and that will be explored here.

Neglect

In healthcare, all nursing associates have a duty of care. This is a legal requirement to provide the best care that meets the expected standard that you can for your patients. If you do not provide that care for your patients and harm is caused, you are neglecting your duty of care, making you negligent. This negligence may be intentional or unintentional, but it results in a patient not receiving proper care. If you are found to be negligent then you could be taken to a hearing of the NMC to discuss whether you should remain on the register of nursing associates or not. The following case study will present a situation where decision-making, best interests and the Bolam test need to be considered.

Case study: Po

You are working a night shift with palliative care patients. One of your patients, Po, aged 13, who lives with a spinal cord injury and needs full care, opens their bowels at 1 a.m. It is very loose and malodorous. When you and a healthcare assistant go to change their pad and bedding you realise that they have diarrhoea and will continue to open their bowels for the next hour. You need to decide whether you should clean and change them every ten minutes or leave them for one hour to fully empty themselves.

Activity 2.2 Reflection

Consider Po's case.

- Which of the two options presented is less harmful to Po?
- By leaving Po, are you being negligent?
- By changing Po every ten minutes are you causing harm through abuse?
- What would a body of your peers decide to do?

An outline answer is provided at the end of the chapter.

Abuse

Abuse in healthcare is causing intentional harm to a person (Adigun et al., 2023). This could be through action or inaction, but the intent is to cause harm. The BBC television programme *Panorama* has exposed many cases over the past few years and here is a summary of some recent stories from the series:

- In October 2022 a Greater Manchester psychiatric hospital was exposed for having a toxic staff culture which led to patients being bullied, taunted and restrained inappropriately. Also, documentation was being falsified, thereby putting patients at risk.
- In October 2012 a home for people with learning difficulties near Bristol was exposed for physically and mentally abusing residents in their care: they were slapped by many members of staff; they had their hair pulled; and they were threatened and intimidated.
- In March 2013 two care homes were exposed for assaulting and abusing their residents both physically and psychologically. This involved multiple members of the healthcare team.

All of the *Panorama* exposures were made possible with secret filming. The filming was undertaken as a last resort after families had raised concerns, and while some staff members pursued these concerns, no action was taken. What seems evident is that there was a lack of transparency and candour in these institutions, with very little thought given to accountability, law or ethics. The cases also revealed a long list of staff members who were either directly involved in the abuse or who were guilty of negligence by not reporting or stopping the abuse. You can view archived episodes of *Panorama* on the BBC website.

Activity 2.3 Work-based learning

- What would you do if you witnessed a colleague using inappropriate language with a patient? This might be swearing at the patient, or calling them names, or generally being mean to them verbally.
- What action would you take?
- What is your role in this situation as a nursing associate?

An outline answer is provided at the end of the chapter.

One of the biggest scandals involved the Mid Staffordshire NHS Foundation Trust and the consequent effect it had on the healthcare services. It led to a public inquiry and the subsequent Francis Report of 2013. The Trust was investigated as it was noted that it had higher than average rates of death for patients admitted via accident and emergency (A & E). The public inquiry took 31 months, and many people were questioned. Ultimately it was determined that the main issue was that the long-term shortage of staff across the Trust led to neglect. It could be argued that this scandal was a case where neglect was sustained for so long that it became abuse, as not meeting the needs of the patients and therefore depriving them of the care that they require is abuse through neglect.

Understanding the theory: neglect and abuse

Neglect is defined as an act of omission in care, leading to potential or actual harm;

Abuse is defined as an act of commission that leads to potential or actual harm (Gonzalez et al., 2023).

The following is an outline of the Mid Staffordshire failures of care:

- higher mortality rates in comparison with other Trusts;
- patients being left in soiled sheets;
- patients not being given food and water;
- leadership not meeting expectations;
- staff members being discouraged from whistleblowing.

The reasons for the Mid Staffordshire failings seem to come from a lack of funding for staff, which led to poor staffing numbers which in turn led to poor care (Francis, 2013). However, this is not an excuse for the level of neglect and abuse that the patients faced. Some staff felt saddened and tried their best with what they had, but other members of staff did not demonstrate compassion towards the patients. There have also been suggestions of bullying and intimidation to stop staff speaking out.

It is important as a nursing associate to be aware of your role in safeguarding and advocating for your patients. Staffing levels are acknowledged as being low and this does cause challenges in delivering care day to day. As a nursing associate you must speak up when you see poor care and follow safeguarding and reporting protocols despite the reasons for the deficit.

Duty of candour, 2018

One of the issues arising from the Mid Staffordshire inquiry was the lack of reporting the poor care and a culture of hiding adverse events. This was due to a number of reasons, including not feeling like a complaint would have any impact and not feeling like it was anyone's responsibility to complain. The duty of candour was brought into effect in 2018 and requires that all registered healthcare professionals are open, honest and transparent with the care that they deliver. If an adverse incident occurs then the person affected (or their representative) must be informed, must receive an apology and must be told what further action is going to take place. This must happen whether a complaint has been made or not. As a nursing associate you are bound under the duty of candour, and you are expected to be honest and open with your own care and the care of others.

Deprivation of Liberty Safeguards 2015

Originally published in 2015, the Deprivation of Liberty Safeguards (DoLS) (SCIE, 2022) is an amendment to the Mental Capacity Act 2005. It links directly to Article 5 of the Human Rights Act. The safeguards are applicable only to people in hospitals and care homes who need to have their freedom restricted in order to protect their own safety: for example, someone who is at risk of leaving the environment and not knowing where they are and therefore becoming lost and putting themselves in danger, or someone who is assessed as being likely to intentionally hurt themselves if they were to leave the environment. There are many ways in which people's freedom is restricted in healthcare. This includes supervision, sedation, physical restraints, and locked wards with codes needed to open the doors. If someone is being deprived of their freedom, then an application must be made for this restriction and authorisation for the restriction needs to be put in place. It needs to be proven that the restrictions are required to protect the patient and safeguard their best interests. This application can take 21 days, which in some situations is not practicable and not safe. Therefore, there is an urgent DoL protocol which allows the deprivation for seven days and which can be extended until the full application is authorised. These safeguards protect vulnerable people from losing their right to justice and fairness in healthcare. It is important to understand the limitations that not having a DoL in place causes as it impacts how the patient can be cared for. For example, if the patient keeps pulling out their nasogastric tube and the nurses want to put mittens on their hands to prevent them from doing this, a DoL must be issued to allow this. If the mittens are put on without the DoL in place, then the patient is being restrained and this could be interpreted as abuse. As a nursing associate you will be involved in safeguarding patients and part of that responsibility is ensuring DoL applications are made appropriately.

Doctrine of double effect

People working in healthcare should never intend to cause harm to their patients. You work in healthcare because you believe in the principle of beneficence (to do good) and non-maleficence (to do no harm), but sometimes we do cause harm and we accept that fact. The doctrine, or rule, of double effect allows foreseen harm to be caused as long as the intended outcome is to do good for the patient. According to Brueck and Sulmasy (2020), this doctrine has some caveats:

- The action being performed must be good within itself.
- The intention of the act is to have a good effect.
- The good act is not caused by the bad effect.
- The bad effect can be rationalised and accounted for.

It is important to accept that we do cause harm to our patients and that is why, when consent is being gained, all information must be given to the patient to ensure that they are prepared for the adverse effects and potential harm. This links with the Bolam test discussed earlier.

Understanding the theory: consent

Consent is intrinsically linked with autonomy, which is intrinsically linked with person-centred care. By explaining to a patient what we want to do we are asking their permission to do this. For the patient to fully understand the procedure it is important that it is described fully. The reason for the procedure must be explained, but along with the positive outcomes it is also important to explain the negative outcomes and the likelihood of each of them. Only when the what, the how, the why and the why nots have been explained can we gain informed consent from a patient. If they understand all the likely outcomes of the procedure and consent to it, then it is acceptable to continue.

Table 2.2 shows three actions that you will perform regularly as a nursing associate that have an intended positive effect on the patient but will also cause harm to the patient. These demonstrate both the Bolam test in healthcare and the doctrine of double effect.

Table 2.2   Examples of actions a nursing associate performs which can cause harm

Act	Intended positive outcome	Acknowledged harm caused
Administering subcutaneous medication.	To alleviate symptoms.	Pain of administration. Adverse side effects. Skin puncture.
Insertion of urinary catheter.	To aid urination.	High risk of infection. Pain and discomfort. Embarrassment.
Repositioning a patient in bed.	To prevent pressure injuries and to promote comfort.	Shearing injuries. Discomfort. Disturbed sleep.

Activity 2.4   Critical thinking

Can you think of examples in your practice where you have knowingly caused harm to your patients even though your intention was to do good?

An outline answer is provided at the end of the chapter.

The NMC's role and responsibilities

The NMC is responsible for ensuring that the high standards expected of healthcare professionals are consistently met. It makes the rules for nurses, midwives and nursing associates through the Code (2018a) as it is the regulatory body. It sets the Standards of Proficiency, and it validates every nursing, midwifery and nursing associate course in the country to ensure it meets the requirements. It considers its main role to be to protect the public and it does this by maintaining high standards for its professionals through regulation of the profession.

NMC hearings

As the regulatory body for nurses, midwives and nursing associates, the NMC investigates when complaints are made or concerns are raised about someone on the register. There is a process that employers must follow and the NMC states that a local investigation and resolution is the best practice, unless the public are at risk. If the employer can intervene quickly and efficiently then that is the most effective way of managing the situation, but if the concern is serious and the public are at risk, then the NMC will get involved in the investigation. Once the NMC has investigated, it can then consider if that person can stay on the register, or if they need a caution, or if they need to be suspended or struck off. Every month the NMC holds fitness to practise hearings which investigate concerns made about nurses, midwives and nursing associates where patients are at risk. The following are reasons to have a NMC hearing:

- Misconduct – falling short of the expectations of the Code.
- Lack of clinical competence – low standards of practice.
- Criminal convictions or cautions – all convictions or cautions must be disclosed.
- Poor health of the practitioner – only if the patients are at risk.
- Poor ability in English – if poor English impacts patient care.
- Determinations by other organisations – if a practitioner is registered with another body who is assessing their fitness to practise, the NMC will also consider it.

Fitness to practise panels are made up of three people: a nurse, midwife or nursing associate (depending on the profession of the person being investigated), an unregistered member of the public and a chair of the panel, who may be a member of the public or a registered professional. One person on the panel needs to be on the same part of the register as the person being investigated. These panel hearings have different outcomes, or sanctions, for the registrant depending on what the decision of the panel is. These are outlined in Table 2.3.

Table 2.3   NMC sanctions (NMC, 2017)

No sanction	It is felt that the person has taken action to improve their clinical practice and no further action is required.
Caution order	This is a warning and can last 1 to 5 years.
Conditions of practice order	The person is still allowed to work, but there are restrictions to their practice. These orders can last 1 to 3 years.
Suspension order	A suspension can last from 1 to 12 months and the person cannot work during this time. A suspension order can be extended if needed.
Striking-off order	The person is removed from the register and cannot work as a registered professional. They can apply to re-join the register after 5 years.

Registrants can also request to be removed from the register and not go through a full hearing. They can re-apply to join after five years if they choose to and undertake a return to practise course. On the NMC website any registrant can be searched for, and their current status is shown with any NMC recognised qualifications and any provisions to their registration.

As well as being answerable to the NMC, nursing associates can also be sued in a civil court. The results of those hearings, and what they are in relation to, need to be considered with their fitness to practise. If a conviction impacts their fitness to practise, then they can be removed from the NMC register.

Ethics

The principles of biomedical ethics (Beauchamp and Childress, 2019) was introduced in Chapter 1. Ethics and the law do not always correlate, but often they do, and they can work together well. Here we will explore a simple case study using the principles of biomedical ethics – autonomy, beneficence, justice and non-maleficence – to consider how UK law supports the decision-making.

Autonomy

Case study: Alice

Alice is a 76-year-old woman admitted to a ward via A & E due to confusion caused by a urine infection. Sian, a nursing associate, has been asked to insert a urinary catheter, but Alice is not giving consent to the procedure. She appears to be rather confused and disorientated. She says that she doesn't know why she has been taken away from her home and wants to go back. She keeps asking for her husband, but he did not come to the hospital with her and her next of kin is her son.

Activity 2.5   Reflection

Consider Alice's case.

- Why might Alice be refusing to consent?
- What steps can Sian take?

We will return to Alice's case later in the chapter.
An outline answer is provided at the end of the chapter.

Respecting the principle of autonomy is to respect your patient's wishes, and that may be asking the practitioner to decide for them, if that is what the patient wants. Respecting autonomy is to give the patient all of the information about any treatment they are to have, including why it is being offered, how it would be administered, the benefits of having it, the adverse effects of having it and the implication of not having it. The patient can then make an informed choice and, even if you do not agree with the choice that is made, you must respect it in order to respect their autonomy. This is true of all patients over the age of 16, unless there is evidence that they are not able to consent. By doing this you are respecting their human rights. Autonomy is intrinsically related to consent. Every patient must be given the opportunity to make an informed decision about their healthcare, and it does not have to be the same decision that the healthcare professionals think they should make. If a healthcare intervention is performed without consent and without respecting autonomy, then assault may have occurred, which is why it is essential that you always obtain consent before performing any interventions on a patient. There are some exceptions to this, however, including in emergency situations, in an operating theatre, if the person is sectioned and needs treatment for their mental health condition or if the person lacks the ability to give consent. If it is felt that someone doesn't have the ability to make a considered decision, then a capacity assessment must be performed to determine whether they have the ability to make the decision or not. This assessment is explained below.

The Mental Capacity Act 2005

The Mental Capacity Act ensures that if healthcare professionals believe that a patient lacks the ability to make an informed decision about their healthcare, an assessment must be done to confirm this. The Act has five principles, which are:

1   A person must be assumed to have capacity unless it is established that they lack capacity.
2   A person is not to be treated as unable to make a decision unless all practicable steps to help them to do so have been taken without success.
3   A person is not to be treated as unable to make a decision merely because they make an unwise decision.
4   An act done, or decision made, under this Act for or on behalf of a person who lacks capacity must be done, or made, in their best interests.
5   Before the act is done, or the decision is made, regard must be had to whether the purpose for which it is needed can be as effectively achieved in a way that is less restrictive of the person's rights and freedom of action

These principles clearly state that if a person is judged to not have capacity, then a decision must be made on their behalf and in their best interests in the way that it is believed they would have chosen if they were able to. According to the Care Quality Commission (2011), assessors of capacity can be any professional involved with the patient. They state that it is the responsibility of everyone involved in decision-making to recognise and assess capacity and that includes nursing associates.

Beneficence

Case study: Alice

Following a capacity assessment by the doctor and a registered nurse, Alice is deemed to not have the capacity to decide whether or not to have the catheter inserted due to her confusion. It is therefore decided that the catheter is to be inserted as it is in her best interests. Sian is asked to proceed with the catheterisation.

Activity 2.6   Reflection

Consider Alice's case.

- How can Alice's autonomy still be respected with the decision that has been made?
- Why was this decision in Alice's best interests?

An outline answer is provided at the end of the chapter.

To administer treatment without the consent of the patient is considered assault in a criminal court. This cannot, by its very nature, be promoting the wellbeing of the patient. However, if an assessment is made and it is agreed that the patient lacks capacity and that with this intervention their health will improve, or their symptoms will reduce, then the intervention is considered to be in their best interests. This is protected in law under the Mental Capacity Act, by the Bolam test and the doctrine of double effect. It is important that you can apply these different laws and assessments in order to ensure you are working in the best interests of the patient. However, considerations also need to be made for what Alice is likely to have consented to when she wasn't confused. Also, there may be less invasive ways to manage the situation until Alice gains the ability to consent following treatment of the urinary tract infection. Alice may not have capacity, but everything should be done to protect her rights as much as possible.

Justice

Case study: Alice

The decision to insert the catheter has been made in Alice's best interests and it is medically advised. However, due to her confusion, she screams and cries when Sian goes to clean her in preparation for the insertion. She calls Sian names and tries to scratch her.

Activity 2.7   Reflection

Consider Alice's case.

- As it is an invasive procedure with risks that she has not consented to, is forcing this catheterisation fair on Alice?
- How can Sian make this process better for her and respect her rights?

An outline answer is provided at the end of the chapter.

Everyone has a right to appropriate treatment under the NHS, even if they are being verbally abusive to the staff. The NHS has a zero-tolerance policy towards abuse to their staff, but patient care is still the priority. If the patient is confused and scared then they need to be cared for accordingly and as a nursing associate you need to communicate with the patient in order to provide comfort and care, even if they are being abusive towards you.

Non-maleficence

Case study: Alice

Alice is very upset and anxious due to having been catheterised, and she is struggling to calm down. Sian goes to talk with her registered nurse about the situation to decide whether the catheterisation caused more harm to Alice than it benefited her.

Activity 2.8   Reflection

Consider Alice's case.

•   Do you think harm was done to Alice?

An outline answer is provided at the end of the chapter.

The intention to do no harm is essential in healthcare. The intention of all care given must be to benefit the patient and be in their best interests. If an undesirable outcome occurs, but the intention was to do good, then your actions are protected in law. As a nursing associate you will be caring for your patients within your scope of practice and within the law in order to promote non-maleficence.

Whistleblowing

While as a nursing associate you are expected to monitor care and report if poor care is being provided, it must be acknowledged that whistleblowing, or raising a concern, can be a daunting thing to do. People are often worried that if they raise concern about another member of staff then they will be treated badly by that person and perhaps the rest of the team. There are cases of people losing their job for whistleblowing. For example, in 2018 a district nurse lost her job when she wanted to initiate whistleblowing procedures regarding low staffing levels which she believed were causing patient deaths. She challenged this decision in court and won the unfair dismissal claim (Baines, 2022). You are protected when you are raising concerns on behalf of a patient and if you do not raise these concerns then you are being negligent in your practice. The duty of candour requires you to whistleblow in order to protect the patients in your care, as does the Code (2018a) and also the Standards of Proficiency for Nursing Associates (NMC, 2018b).

Chapter summary

This chapter has explored some of the laws that govern the day-to-day work of healthcare professionals. It has considered where ethics and law work well together, and where they sometimes don't. It has also looked at cases where the law was not abided by, and patients suffered. Professional guidelines for nursing associates were also considered.

Activities: Brief outline answers

Activity 2.1

What is true according to UK law?

It is a legal requirement that you help to save a drowning child.	False	There is no legal obligation to help this child if you choose not to. There is a moral and ethical obligation to assist if you are able to.
It is against the law to park on double red lines.	True	No stopping, waiting, loading or dropping off or picking up passengers on a double red line is permitted other than licensed taxis and blue badge holders.
It is against the law to kill a swan.	True	This is an offence under the Salmon Act of 1986. All swans are the property of the monarch and must not be killed.
It is a legal requirement that you must always try to prevent someone from committing suicide.	False	Suicide was decriminalised in the Suicide Act of 1961 so it is not a crime to kill yourself. You are not legally obliged to stop someone killing themselves. However, it is against the law to help someone to kill themselves in any way and this is punishable with up to 14 years in prison.
It is against the law to drink alcohol and drive a car.	False	It is not against the law to drink and drive, but there are strict limits as to how much can be consumed and if these are exceeded it does become a criminal offence.
It is against the law to smoke in a car with a child present.	True	The Children and Families Act of 2014 made it illegal to smoke in a private car with a passenger under the age of 18.

Activity 2.2

Both of the options for this patient have negative elements. By changing Po every ten minutes you will cause trauma and discomfort and it will be very tiring for Po and for you. By leaving Po for one hour you risk excoriation from leaving faeces in situ. You need to be very conscious of time and ensure you don't leave Po for longer than required. In situations like this there is no correct answer. You need to decide the best course of action at the time, weighing up the consequences of each action.

Activity 2.3

Your role as a nursing associate is to protect and advocate for your patients. The duty of candour instructs you to be open and transparent about incorrect or inappropriate care.

You have a duty of care to your patients to provide the best care possible , and a member of staff verbally abusing patients is not the best care available. If you witness poor care you must report it to the appropriate person, complete the appropriate paperwork and apologise to the patient or their family for the poor care.

Activity 2.4

A lot of clinical procedures that you perform have the potential to cause harm to your patients, for example, the administration of medication, repositioning someone or breaking bad news. Moreover, there is the possibility that any errors or mistakes that you make will potentially cause harm to a patient. It is not uncommon to harm patients – hopefully only in minor ways – but if the intention is to work in what is considered to be their best interests, then your actions are acceptable.

Activity 2.5

We know that Alice is confused, and a urine infection can be the cause of that, so she needs a capacity assessment to decide if at that time she has the capacity to refuse the catheter. If she has capacity, then the team needs to understand why she is refusing. She may have had a bad experience in the past; she may have heard horrible stories from friends; she may have been abused; or she may simply be scared and confused. It is part of the nursing associate's role to communicate with her and reassure her and to help her understand why she needs to have the catheter.

Activity 2.6

It can be argued that once the catheter is inserted then Alice will be in less pain and she will be less symptomatic, which is in her best interests and therefore justifies the catheterisation. Once Alice is assessed to have capacity again, she can then have the catheter removed if that is what she wants. Another option could be to find a less invasive procedure until the infection has started to subside and Alice starts to regain capacity and see what her decision is then. This would protect Alice's autonomy as much as possible.

Activity 2.7

As the treatment is in Alice's best interests medically, and she lacks capacity, it is fair that she has the treatment. She needs reassurance and comfort and not to be rushed through the procedure. Healthcare professionals do not know what she has been through in her life and it is important to remember that. It is important that she is catheterised even if she is verbally or physically abusive to staff, and staff must be patient and understanding.

Activity 2.8

The intention of the catheterisation was to reduce discomfort for Alice. If she was communicated with throughout the procedure and she was made as comfortable as possible, then her best interests were promoted by this action. However, it cannot be stated that no harm was caused during this procedure as Alice is clearly upset and distressed by being catheterised and this needs to be documented fully.

Further reading

Cribb, A and Tingle, J (2014) *Nursing Law and Ethics* (4th edn). Oxford: Wiley-Blackwell.

This book explores nursing-focused legal and ethical issues. It utilises case studies to apply the theory to practice.

Herring, J (2022) *Medical law and Ethics* (9th edn). Oxford: Oxford University Press.

This book considers medical issues that arise in practice from a focus on the complex issues that arise in practice.

GOV.UK (2015) *Equality Act 2010: Guidance.* Available at: **www.gov.uk/guidance/ equality-act-2010-guidance**

Information and guidance on the Equality Act 2010, including age discrimination and public sector Equality Duty.

GOV.UK (2023) *Mental Capacity Act: Making Decisions.* Available at: **www.gov.uk/ government/collections/mental-capacity-act-making-decisions**

Guidance on how to make decisions under the 2005 Mental Capacity Act.

Useful websites

www.bbc.co.uk/programmes/b006t14n

Watch old episodes of the BBC programme *Panorama*.

www.equalityhumanrights.com

The official website of the Equality and Human Rights Commission, which enforces the Equality Act 2010.

www.parliament.uk/about/how/laws/

The UK Parliament's guide to how laws are made.

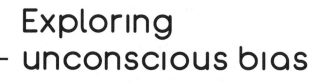

Exploring unconscious bias

Chapter

3

NMC STANDARDS OF PROFICIENCY FOR NURSING ASSOCIATES

This chapter will address the following platforms and proficiencies:

Platform 1: Being an accountable professional

1.3   understand the importance of courage and transparency and apply the Duty of Candour, recognising and reporting any situations, behaviours or errors that could result in poor care outcomes

1.4   demonstrate an understanding of, and the ability to, challenge or report discriminatory behaviour

1.5   understand the demands of professional practice and demonstrate how to recognise signs of vulnerability in themselves or their colleagues and the action required to minimise risks to health

1.15   take responsibility for continuous self-reflection, seeking and responding to support and feedback to develop professional knowledge and skills

1.16   act as an ambassador for their profession and promote public confidence in health and care services

Platform 5: Improving safety and quality of care

5.9   recognise uncertainty and demonstrate an awareness of strategies to develop resilience in themselves. Know how to seek support to help deal with uncertain situations

Platform 6: Contributing to integrated care

6.5   identify when people need help to facilitate equitable access to care, support and escalate concerns appropriately

Chapter aims

After reading this chapter, you will be able to:

- demonstrate an understanding of unconscious bias;
- develop an awareness of your own bias;
- understand the negative impact that bias can have on healthcare;
- explore different methods to minimise negative actions that arise from bias.

'Everybody is a genius. But if you judge a fish by its ability to climb a tree, it will live its whole life believing that it is stupid.' (Albert Einstein, 1952, quoted in Kelly, 2004)

Introduction

Unconscious bias has been part of the NHS mandatory training for some years now. This training was introduced to minimise decisions being made about people based on certain characteristics like their race, looks or accent, to name but a few. The training asks you to consider any opinions you may have based on certain characteristics like the ones mentioned, but the training is quite generic. This chapter will help you understand unconscious bias in a more in-depth manner to help you practise in a more equitable way.

Nursing associates are expected to advocate for all the people that they are caring for, but sometimes there are unknown internal barriers which impact the way in which care is delivered. The UK is a vibrant multicultural country, but different cultures bring different experiences, and these experiences can be both positive and negative. These experiences can lead to judgements and prejudices being incorporated into everyday care, which is why it is important to be aware of them.

What is unconscious bias?

Unconscious bias is described as the associations that people make with certain characteristics that affect the way that they treat people (Marcelin et al., 2019). Judgements can be made very quickly and are often unfairly based on random criteria without looking at other aspects of that person. They are called unconscious bias because, until you look at yourself and reflect on judgements made, you are not aware that you have them.

Activity 3.1   Critical thinking

Consider the following questions and reflect on your initial thoughts about each of them.

- Are you surprised when you see a mixed-race couple?
- Do you expect a pilot to be male or female?
- Do you expect a nurse to be male or female?

- Do you expect a doctor to be male or female?
- In a male–female couple, who do you think makes the meals?
- In a male–female couple, who do you think should wash the clothes?
- In a male–female couple, who do you think should put the bins out?
- What colour clothes do you think girls and boys should wear?
- Do you consider James to be a boy's name or a girl's name?

An outline answer is provided at the end of the chapter.

It must be noted that not all judgemental behaviour is actually unconscious. Some of it is very conscious and planned and used with malicious intent. This chapter is not looking at that type of judgemental behaviour; it is focusing on the unintentional biases and accompanying microaggressions that we deal with every day.

The phenomenon of unconscious bias was originally highlighted in job interviews where there was clear preference given to certain applicants while others were excluded from the same opportunities (Sippet, 2015). This could be based on the applicant's gender, ethnicity, size or age, among other values. The judgements were not about the ability to do the job, but about a random, inconsequential variable which the applicant could not change. In healthcare we would like to think that judgemental behaviour is not practised, but unconscious bias is not something that people can control, unless they have a full understanding of their own limitations. Gopal et al. (2021) conducted a literature review on bias in clinical decision-making and found a high incidence of it. They argue that there is no effective debiasing strategy in place in healthcare and that awareness alone is not enough to counter it.

Where does unconscious bias come from?

The question of how we get our biases is a challenging one. People are not born with prejudice; we learn our biases from the people and the world around us – our parents, our carers, our teachers, our friends, the television programmes that we watch, the books that we read and the people that we listen to. As we grow up, we are subjected to views and opinions that become part of our own personalities and form our own opinions about people we may have never come across personally.

Types of bias

There are many different types of bias and different ways to be judgemental. A lot of information about unconscious bias comes from employment data, but the biases are relevant in all elements of life and are easily related to healthcare. Various websites list different types and different amounts of bias. Table 3.1 identifies ten different forms of bias that are listed by the National School of Healthcare Science (NHS England, 2022). However, there are sources that list up to 19 different types, so this list is not exhaustive.

Before you think of how these biases affect healthcare delivery, think of your own life and situations where you have experienced such biases in action and consider whether there was a negative or positive outcome from this. A lot of our relationships are formed on the basis of our instinctive reactions towards people, and we tend to eliminate those with whom we do not feel a

Table 3.1   Types of bias

Affinity bias	Affinity bias is sometimes called similarity bias and is where people prefer the company of people from similar backgrounds and have similar interests. Day to day that isn't an issue as long as it doesn't impact on the way that you treat people who don't look like you or don't have a similar background to you.
Ageism	Age is a protected characteristic, but age bias affects people every day. For example, if you, as a student, are working with a staff nurse younger than you, a lot of patients will assume that you are the senior practitioner based purely on your age.
Anchor bias	Anchor bias is relying on the first piece of information you hear about something and not taking into consideration things that you learn later on. This could be about a person or a situation, or anything else.
Attribution bias	Attribution bias is where people are judged, and assumptions are made, about why someone is behaving in a certain way. These assumptions are not reflecting the individual person but are based on the preconceived ideas that we have about them.
Beauty bias	Beauty bias is simply preferring someone who is attractive and giving them preferential treatment over someone who you don't find as nice to look at. We must allocate ourselves according to need, not according to how much we like the patient.
Confirmation bias	Confirmation bias is the process of choosing to only hear a certain piece of information that confirms a previously made opinion. For example, consider the patient who is asking for strong painkillers due to a severe headache, but is refused based on their colour and the opinion that they are drug addicts. Their information is not heard, just certain elements of it which confirm 'drug-seeking behaviour'. Instead of assessing the patient fully, it is assumed that they are simply seeking drugs.
Conformity bias	Conformity bias is when your opinion changes based on what you are told, not on what you actually think. Patient handover is a situation in which this can occur, and it is important to not make judgemental comments in handover to reduce the risk of prejudice.
Contrast effect	The contrast effect is where judgements are made based on what others experience. Patients and relatives sometimes do this by comparing the level of care they receive in comparison to another patient, without considering the different care needs.
Gender bias	Gender bias is making assumptions about a person based on their gender. This can be positive or negative. An example is when a judgement is made regarding what job is suitable for what person based purely on their gender, not on their personal abilities or preferences. It's the idea of some jobs being 'women's jobs' and some jobs being 'men's jobs'. In healthcare, for example, nurses are largely thought of as being female and doctors male, although obviously that isn't true.
Halo effect	The halo effect is when someone is given preferential treatment based on one bit of information, like the university they graduated from as opposed to their ability to do the job.
Name bias	In employment data there has been a lot of evidence showing that a person with an English sounding name will be given a job opportunity rather than someone with a non-English sounding name.

connection. Tsipursky and McRaney (2020) explore how trusting our gut feeling is instinctive, but that it isn't always accurate. Relationships break down despite your gut feeling telling you that person is perfect for you. Friends argue and drift apart, which might make you question your instincts. The same is true of your patients. As a nursing associate you might instinctively warm towards a certain patient because they remind you of someone you care about, or you feel a connection with them. You might struggle to connect with a different patient although you can't necessarily pinpoint as to why. This is your gut instinct or, in other words, your unconscious bias. The eventual outcome of trusting your gut is the impact this may have on the care that you deliver. Recognising this in yourself and seeing it in the rest of the multidisciplinary team is essential for good care delivery.

When considering the issue of unconscious bias, you need to remember that the patients and their families also have these feelings. White and Chanoff (2011) discuss the fact that patients feel more trust if the person looking after them is from the same culture as them. They instantly feel more comfortable, more understood and more seen. This means that communication is better in this situation. This is not practicable in healthcare, which is why it is important that healthcare professionals have an understanding of different cultures in order to understand the needs and fears of them better.

Unconscious bias and the protected characteristics of the Equality Act 2010

The biases shown in Table 3.1 can be linked directly to the nine protected characteristics of the Equality Act and Table 3.2 considers different case studies that provide examples of how each characteristic can have a bias applied.

Table 3.2 Unconscious bias and the protected characteristics

Characteristic	Types of bias that could be applied	Example case study
Age	Ageism, attribution bias, beauty bias, halo effect	A 19-year-old patient has been diagnosed with a brain tumour and has been offered full treatment with a good chance of success. However, he has refused the treatment and would rather be allowed to die. The team wants to speak with his family and have him assessed for capacity as they think he doesn't fully understand the situation due to his age.
Disability	Attribution bias, beauty bias, halo effect	A nursing assistant is doing a bank shift on a ward they are not familiar with. A woman in her mid-twenties appears in a wheelchair. It is not visiting hours. She is wearing her own clothes, and the nursing associate asks her if she is a patient on the ward. She gets offended and informs them quite rudely that she is in fact a doctor and is there to see patients, not to be a patient.
Gender reassignment	Confirmation bias, attribution bias	A patient who identifies as non-binary is admitted to a ward. The staff continue to use gender-based pronouns for this patient throughout their admission. The patient becomes upset at first and then angry and states they are going to make a formal complaint.
Race	Name bias, confirmation bias, attribution bias	A man presents to A & E one Saturday night complaining of a severe headache. He is told to go home and sleep it off. It is assumed he is seeking drugs. The man is 22 years old and he is Black. On Sunday morning he is admitted via ambulance as he was unresponsive at home.

(Continued)

Table 3.2 (Continued)

Characteristic	Types of bias that could be applied	Example case study
Marriage and civil partnership	Affinity bias	A 28-year-old married woman is a patient in the maternity department. She is 32 weeks pregnant and has been bleeding, so has been admitted for observation. She is understandably rather anxious. She has been reassured multiple times that the baby's father can visit from 9 a.m.
		A female visitor arrives to support the patient and she is asked if she knows when the patient's husband will be visiting. The visitor has to explain that the patient doesn't have a husband; she has a wife, and she is that wife.
Pregnancy and maternity	Affinity bias, confirmation bias, age bias	A woman aged 23 has presented to her GP, asking to be referred for a full hysterectomy. She doesn't want to have children and she has endometriosis which causes her a lot of pain. She has full capacity and wants a hysterectomy. The GP is not happy to make this referral as they believe that the woman is too young to make this decision.
Religion or belief	Affinity bias, name bias, confirmation bias	A complaint is issued against a nurse who told every patient she saw that she would pray for them. She meant this with only good intentions, but some patients and relatives took offence. She has been doing this for her whole career of 36 years and it is only now that a complaint has been made.
Sex	Gender bias, confirmation bias, age bias	A patient on the ward is being reviewed by the urological surgical team. The patient gets angry and wants to speak to the consultant. He will not believe that the doctor speaking to him is the consultant as the doctor is female and looks to be in her forties.
Sexual orientation	Attribution bias	A woman is in hospital requiring pre-assessment health checks. The nursing associate assigned to look after her is wearing a rainbow badge signifying support for LGBTQIA+. The patient asks if this nursing associate is gay, and she confirms that she is. The patient asks for a different member of staff to look after her as she doesn't want the nursing associate to be attracted to her.

Activity 3.2   Decision-making

For each example listed in Table 3.2, consider which types of bias were applied and what, as a nursing associate, you could do in the given situation.

An outline answer is provided at the end of the chapter.

Table 3.2 only provides a brief list of examples of the ways in which you might encounter unconscious bias. There are many more situations that occur that you may have experienced or witnessed. It is particularly important to recognise the ways in which unconscious bias might affect the protected characteristics.

Understanding unconscious bias is an important step in improving your work as a nursing associate.

Minimising the impact of unconscious bias

Unconscious bias is clearly a common occurrence, but it is not acceptable to ignore it as bias can lead to oppression. The first step to minimise the impact of unconscious bias is to recognise it. You need to recognise it both in yourself and in others (Noon, 2018) and you need to verbalise it when you do see it as the person perpetuating it may not have had the training that you have had. That can be challenging, but without verbalising it change will not happen.

As a nursing associate you are well placed to manage your own unconscious bias. Simple personal strategies to reduce your bias include making no assumptions, keeping communication open and listening to the person in front of you before making decisions about them. Marcelin et al. (2019) state that people need to take three steps to counter their own bias. These three steps are:

- Be aware of your own biases.
- Be systematic in assuring you are not applying your biases.
- Be open to new experiences in order to grow and develop.

Microaggressions

Microaggression is a term used for everyday remarks and actions that express a prejudicial attitude toward a member of a socially marginalised group. Like unconscious bias, people may not be aware they are exhibiting such behaviour until they engage in self-reflection. Microaggressions can be very hurtful but often the people being subjected to microaggressions appear to ignore them (Alabi, 2015), which can make them seem acceptable. There are some actions or exchanges that could be interpreted in different ways, and although they may be well-intentioned and not meant to be malicious, if these actions are interpreted as microaggressions, then that is what they are.

Other ways to describe a microaggression include subtle acts of exclusion or a micro-assault. They are words or actions that make it clear that someone is 'different' and excludes them. As a nursing associate, assumptions about people must never be made, be they positive or negative. Open-ended questions should be used when assessing someone and your own opinion and feelings should not be a part of the care that you deliver. Table 3.3 provides some examples of microaggressive statements set specifically against the nine protected characteristics.

Table 3.3 Examples of microaggressions and the nine protected characteristics

Nine protected characteristics	Examples of microaggressions (not an exhaustive list)
Age	'She is old', 'the elderly'.
Disability	'That is so lame'.
Gender reassignment	Deadnaming someone.
Marriage and civil partnership	'When are you getting married?'
Pregnancy and maternity	'When are you going to have children? Your biological clock is ticking'.
Race	'I don't think of you as Black'.
Religion or belief	'Of course, Jews are good with money'.
Sex	'Sweetheart', 'little lady', 'man up'.
Sexual orientation	'You don't look gay'.

There are many other examples of microaggressions that you hear or say every day.

As a nursing associate it is essential that inappropriate behaviour is recognised and highlighted to hopefully eradicate derogatory attitudes in the future. You will witness microaggressions towards your patients or members of your team and you need to consider how you will respond to them.

Chapter summary

This chapter has explored the notion of unconscious bias. It has explored different types of bias and how they impact the nine protected characteristics of the Equality Act. It has also highlighted the importance of the role of the nursing associate in protecting all of the patients who are in need of care.

Activities: Brief outline answers

Activity 3.1

If you have certain instinctive answers to any of these questions, then you have unconscious biases. They come from various places and they do not always lead to discrimination as long as you are aware of them and can challenge them within yourself. You will have instinctive reactions to people and situations, but you need to decide whether they are appropriate or not in your healthcare role and try to change your instincts to be more inclusive.

Activity 3.2

Table 3.2 gave unconscious bias examples to demonstrate situations you may find yourself in. You must remember that all patients deserve respect at all times. No one should be judged on how they look or by your own personal beliefs about different groups of people.

Age

Once a patient reaches the age of 18, they can make decisions about their healthcare without the need of input from their family members. To assume that a patient does not understand the implications of their decision is patronising and ageist. The team cannot discuss the situation with the family without permission from the patient first. As a nursing associate you can take the time to talk with the patient and explore why they have made a particular decision and thereby participate in protecting their autonomy.

Disability

To assume that someone in a wheelchair must be a patient or a visitor of a patient is inappropriate. Healthcare is changing and there is no reason why someone in a wheelchair couldn't be a healthcare professional. The medicalisation and perception bias of somebody with altered physical ability is common and it is offensive. Instead of making assumptions, greet someone you don't know by introducing yourself as a nursing associate, asking their name and asking if you can help them.

Gender reassignment

People have the right to identify with any gender they choose or indeed not identify with a gender at all. The use of gender-based pronouns is becoming less advisable until the preference of a person is known. Person-centred care means working with the patients and meeting their personal needs. This can only be achieved with effective communication, which nursing associates are well placed to promote.

Race

The assumption that a young Black person is seeking drugs when presenting to A & E is not unusual. There are many cases to be found that show young people, particularly Black men, are not being assessed properly due to the assumption that they are seeking drugs. This perception bias is discriminatory. This isn't an exclusively UK issue. Hoffman et al. (2016) conducted a study in America which showed that 50 per cent of people felt that people of African American heritage were thought to experience pain differently and were therefore routinely under-treated for pain in comparison to their white counterparts. There is no reason to think this; it is not based on biology or science.

As a nursing associate, your role is to advocate for the patient and be the voice that they don't always have in order to promote person-centred care.

Marriage and civil partnership

The assumption that every couple is heterosexual is uninformed and it excludes many people. Same-sex marriage is legal in this country and healthcare professionals should never assume who someone's partner is. This example of anchor bias abuses both marriage and sexual orientation. Incorrectly assuming such a thing alienates the patient and reduces the trust between the patient and the healthcare staff. As a nursing associate you should always communicate with the patient and ask open questions to allow them to speak freely, and this will promote a positive therapeutic relationship.

Pregnancy and maternity

The assumption that every woman will want to have children is common but inappropriate: there are many who do not want to have children. In this situation, as long as all information is given to the patient it can be easy to determine whether that patient has the capacity to make this decision. As a nursing associate you can talk with the patient to help work through any concerns that the GP has. Communication-skills training is really useful and worth pursuing as it will help you in your career as a nursing associate.

Religion

Everybody has the right to hold religious beliefs and the Equality Act makes it clear that this also includes the right to not have a religious belief. To impose your personal beliefs onto others is a breach of the Code (NMC, 2018a). Ideally, the nurse should be spoken to and the issue explained. Although she means no harm, if her words cause offence then they are not comforting the patient. Sometimes the thought of approaching a nurse of a higher grade than you to criticise her behaviour is intimidating, but the needs of the patient must come first. Find a way to communicate which causes the least amount of harm to maintain good working relationships.

Sex

Patients have perceptions of what a consultant should look like, but these perceptions are being challenged every day. This perception bias and gender bias is a common occurrence and, hopefully, as more diversity in professional roles in healthcare becomes apparent, such biases will start to disappear. The opportunity to become a nursing associate is open to anyone of any age and any gender, and this is a positive aspect of the role as it will help to reduce gender bias.

Sexual orientation

Patients do have the right to refuse care from certain people, but to base that decision on someone's sexuality is against the Equality Act. As a nursing associate you can reassure the patient that staff will always be professional, and that a chaperone can be provided for personal care if required.

Useful websites

www.nonprofitready.org/unconscious-bias-training

This website offers free unconscious bias training.

https://training.nottingham.ac.uk/Public/Unconscious-Bias-Workbook.pdf

A workbook to help you assess your bias.

https://asana.com/resources/unconscious-bias-examples

A website to look at different unconscious bias categories.

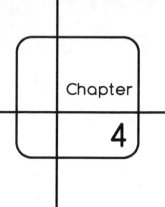

Chapter 4

Exploring diversity

NMC STANDARDS OF PROFICIENCY FOR NURSING ASSOCIATES

The chapter will address the following platforms and proficiencies:

Platform 1: Being an accountable professional

1.4   demonstrate an understanding of, and the ability to, challenge or report discriminatory behaviour

1.11   provide, promote, and where appropriate advocate for, non-discriminatory, person-centred and sensitive care at all times. Reflect on people's values and beliefs, diverse backgrounds, cultural characteristics, language requirements, needs and preferences, taking account of any need for adjustments

Platform 2: Promoting health and preventing ill health

2.3   describe the principles of epidemiology, demography, and genomics and how these may influence health and wellbeing outcomes

2.4   understand the factors that may lead to inequalities in health outcomes

2.5   understand the importance of early years and childhood experiences and the possible impact on life choices, mental, physical and behavioural health and wellbeing

2.6   understand and explain the contribution of social influences, health literacy, individual circumstances, behaviours and lifestyle choices to mental, physical and behavioural health outcomes

Platform 5: Improving safety and quality of care

5.8   understand when to seek appropriate advice to manage a risk and avoid compromising quality of care and health outcomes

5.9   recognise uncertainty, and demonstrate an awareness of strategies to develop resilience in themselves. Know how to seek support to help deal with uncertain situations

Chapter aims

After reading this chapter, you will be able to:

- understand diversity in England;
- understand the challenges of resource allocation;
- understand the importance of the UK Census;
- identify specific health needs for specific ethnic groups.

Understanding the theory: key terminology

Health inequality – unavoidable and unfair differences in health between groups of people.

Diversity – the differences that make a person an individual.

Demographics – the use of statistics about a geographical area to identify needs.

Integrated care boards – replaced clinical commissioning groups in 2022. The integrated care boards (ICBs) are responsible for managing the health of a geographical area and the budget for it.

'Diversity is the one true thing we all have in common ... celebrate it every day.'
(Author unknown, although it is often attributed to Winston Churchill)

Introduction

This chapter will consider the complex topic of diversity and explore the different factors that make up a person's cultural identity. It will describe diversity in the UK based on the results of the 2022 Census. It will look at regional differences and how these impact on healthcare delivery in relation to some of the protected characteristics of the Equality Act of 2010. The chapter will consider specific ethnic health needs and the challenges faced by the healthcare providers.

Diversity is the practice of including people from different social and ethnic backgrounds, and understanding that people are different and that no two people are exactly the same. Everyone has an individual identity which is developed through many different factors and experiences. As a nursing associate you will care for people from different backgrounds and cultures. However, the amount of diversity you will see is dependent on where you are working due to geographical diversity. This will be explored further in this chapter. Diversity is intrinsically linked with equity. To meet the needs of all people in your care you need to understand the differences in order to adapt the care being given and provide person-centred equitable care.

Anca and Aragon (2018) describe three types of diversity:

- demographic (gender, race, religion);
- experiential (lifestyle);
- cognitive (learning styles).

They argue that each person's culture is based on all of these factors. Activity 4.1 asks you to consider the different factors that make up your personal culture.

Activity 4.1   Reflection

Consider how you identify asking yourself the following questions:

- Where do you live?
- Where were you born?
- Where does your family live?
- How old are you?
- What language(s) do you speak?
- What religion do you follow, if any?
- What gender do you identify as?
- Is that the gender you were born with?
- Are you married? (Or in a long-term relationship?)
- Do you have any children?
- What kind of food do you eat?
- What kind of music do you listen to?
- Do you celebrate any special days or festivals?
- Do you have any hobbies?
- What kind of a learner are you?
- Do you have any physical or cognitive diagnoses?

As this activity is a personal reflection, no outline answer is provided at the end of the chapter.

The exercise in Activity 4.1 illustrates the fact that a person's identity is complex and multifaceted. It isn't simply about where a person lives or what religion they practise, for example, but it is a mixture of all the different elements that make a person who they are.

In 1986 Milton Bennett designed a scale of cultural competence (see Figure 4.1 and Table 4.1), which consists of six stages which take you on a journey from ethnocentrism (where a person's personal culture is understood as being the 'normal' culture and everything else is 'abnormal') to ethnorelativism (where a person understands many different cultures and knows that their own culture is one of many) (Bennett, 1986).

Denial	Defence	Minimisation	Acceptance	Adaption	Integration
Ethnocentrism		➝			Ethnorelativism

Figure 4.1   Bennett's scale of cultural competence (1986)

Table 4.1   Explanation of the stages of Bennett's scale

Denial	This stage is when a person doesn't recognise cultural differences or discounts them as being irrelevant.
Defence	This stage is seeing different cultures in a polarised way with racial stereotyping, such as stating that immigrants steal all the jobs or all Black men are criminals.
Minimisation	This stage is when someone doesn't recognise cultural differences and claims everyone is the same. A statement like 'I don't see colour' is an example of minimisation.
Acceptance	This stage involves the recognition of differences between different cultures. There may also be an increase of interest in other cultures at this stage in order to broaden knowledge and understanding.
Adaptation	This stage occurs when cultural differences are understood and adjustments made to accommodate them. This does not mean that the person has to leave their own culture and adopt a new culture; it is being able to adapt to the different needs of various cultures.
Integration	This is when a person's identity incorporates different beliefs and values from various cultures. It is to be multicultural as a person and understand how different cultures can work together and learn and grow from those differences.

The following case study is a practical if rather simple example of the stages of cultural competence.

Case study: Cultural competence

You are working on a ward and there is an international recruitment drive. Nurses are employed from overseas and English is not their first language, and many of them are devout Catholics, which you are not. You are working with a group of them, and they are struggling to understand medical terminology and to keep up with the fast-paced conversations that include local colloquialisms.

Denial – You carry on as normal, stating that in England everyone's the same and no changes should be made to accommodate newcomers in the workplace. If someone chooses to come to England to work, then they should be able to manage.

↓   ↓

Defence – You become annoyed at the nurses not being able to understand conversations well and believe that all foreign nurses can't be bothered to learn English properly and that they only come here to earn more money and use the NHS. They also prevent English nurses from getting jobs.

↓   ↓

Minimisation – You believe that as they are working as nurses they should adjust and be seen as nurses and their ethnicity and cultural background is irrelevant and should not be considered.

↓   ↓

Acceptance – You are interested in the differences between your own culture and the culture of the overseas nurses as you can see that different cultures may have different needs that should be met.

↓   ↓

Adaptation – You understand the cultural differences between your own culture and that of the overseas nurses and you adjust your own language and habits to accommodate the needs of others. You also see the strengths in some of the differences and the benefits of many of them.

↓   ↓

Integration – You understand different cultures and any requirements that they may have, and you incorporate them into your everyday life without conscious thought. For example, you explain things that you say, and you don't use jargon or colloquial language and you don't blaspheme, as that can offend your colleagues.

Activity 4.2 considers the practical elements of cultural competence in a hospital environment. It demonstrates some of the challenges that need to be overcome to make a hospital ward integrate a variety of cultures.

Activity 4.2   Critical thinking

Consider a hospital environment where you have worked. How culturally competent was it? Was it adapted to multiple cultures, or had it integrated multiple cultures? Consider the following things:

1.   How diverse was the menu? Did it cater for:

- Meat-eaters?
- Meat-eaters with halal or kosher requirements?
- Vegetarians?
- Vegans?

2.   How easy was it for religious guidance to be provided for a variety of faiths? How quickly could a religious leader get to the hospital to provide support for the patient? How might a delay have impacted the patient and their family?

3.   Consider the signs on the walls. What language were they in? How might this have impacted the patient and their family and friends?

4.   What was the visiting policy where you were? Were there time restrictions? Were the numbers of visitors restricted? How might these restrictions have affected the family and friends of the patient, and the patient themself?

As this activity is a personal reflection, no outline answer is provided at the end of the chapter.

Every ward should be as inclusive as possible with signs in as many different languages as possible on display. Religious leaders should be local and able to come to see patients as soon as possible; finding their contact details should also be easily done. Calendars with different religious festivals could be displayed on all wards to help the staff to understand the significance of certain dates for different people.

Visiting hours impact families and communities in different ways. Some people want all of their family with them, which can be challenging in a busy ward environment. Some relatives will disturb other patients while being a soothing presence for their loved one. This can cause unrest in a ward, and this is not a good healing environment. It is important to try to find a solution that is beneficial for all parties, but sometimes that is not possible and the decision may need to rely on the policies of the clinical area.

As a nursing associate you should aim to be on the ethnorelativism end of the Bennett scale in order to look after your patients with equity and you should be able to integrate cultures into your lifestyle by expanding your knowledge and understanding of them. Some specific cultural health beliefs will be discussed in Chapter 8.

There are various self-evaluation tools online to work through to reflect upon your own feelings and actions with cultures that are different from your own. The main message to take home from them seems to be to keep reflecting on how you feel and self-evaluating your actions in order to ensure you are as culturally competent as you can be. Your competence will be limited by your unconscious bias, so it is important to keep reflecting to reduce your own bias.

The Census

Once every ten years, the population of England and Wales is asked to complete a survey which asks questions about households and the people living in them. England and Wales are divided into ten separate geographical areas and this provides a snapshot of the demographics of each area of the two countries. The data is used to help the government make decisions regarding schools, healthcare provision and fund allocation. This information enables us to understand the different needs in these parts of the country and provide care and services that are appropriate for the population living in those areas.

The Census asks people 41 questions, and it has been a legal requirement to complete it since the Census Act of 1920. Not completing it or falsifying information is punishable with a fine of up to £1,000. The questions are a mixture of simple and multiple choice and not all are mandatory. The questions are about both the individual and the household. Simple questions tackle topics like name, age, sex, sexual orientation and marital status and ask about people's ethnicity, religion, country of birth, national identity and language. The Census also asks specific health questions about how that individual is feeling in general, whether they have any mental health conditions or physical conditions that have lasted, or may last, more than 12 months. It also asks if there are caring responsibilities for that person. It asks about education level and job status. The household questions look at the dynamics of the household, including how many people live there and what their relationship is to the individual completing the Census. It asks individual questions about each person living in that household, including the age, gender, ethnic group, national identity, religion, sexual orientation, health conditions, education level and job status and role. The questions include the protected characteristics of the Equality Act of 2010.

Through the Census it is possible to see the ethnic diversity in each of the ten areas in England and Wales. The Census shows clearly that London is the most ethnically diverse area in England and Wales, and the North East is the least ethnically diverse. However, it also shows that there is ethnic diversity in every region of England, which is important to remember. In London, seeing people with different-coloured skin is a constant occurrence. But in some small towns in the North East, for example, it will be unusual to see people from a non-white background, which may have an impact on access to healthcare and on healthcare delivery. You can see the data on the Office for National Statistics (ONS) website.

The Census is important as it helps to direct resource allocation in the NHS. Central money is divided among the ICBs to allocate the funds in their locality. With the information from the Census, it is possible for the ICBs to meet the needs of their particular population.

When considering sexuality in England and Wales, the Census states that London has the highest percentage of LGBTQIA+ people in all of England and Wales and the North East of England has the lowest number. It is then logical to assume that London will have the highest quantity of facilities for LGBTQIA+ people and that London ICBs will allocate more funds for specific health services for LGBTQIA+ people than an area which has a low percentage of this population like the North East (ONS, 2022). These might include facilities such as mental health support services, housing services, anti-violence and abuse charities, support groups, gender reassignment surgical centres and other services that specialise in supporting LGBTQIA+ people at every stage of their journey. It does make sense for London to devote more funds than other areas, but the Census clearly shows that there are LGBTQIA+ people all over England and Wales, albeit in lower numbers. The areas with a low percentage of LGBTQIA+ people may devote less money to specialised services, which can be isolating for people in this group. This may mean that they don't access healthcare support when they need to, which has an impact on their health and wellbeing.

Ethnic-specific situations

There are some conditions and illnesses that, although anyone from any background can have them, will be more prevalent in certain ethnicities. It is important to know about the ethnic demographics of the area in which you are working as that will inform you of some of the illnesses you need to know about to meet the needs of your diverse patients. Examples of such conditions are type II diabetes, sickle cell disease and coronary heart disease.

Type II diabetes

Type II diabetes has a high incidence rate in people who are South Asian, Black African, and African Caribbean and it develops at a younger age than in people from a white ethnic background. The reasons are not fully known but it is suggested that it may be due to how fat is stored in people from those ethnic backgrounds (Hanif and Susarla, 2018). Though it is recognised by the NHS that a *healthy body mass index is between 20 and 25* (NHS, 2023), for people from a non-white ethnic background, it is suggested that their BMI is kept at less than 23. This information is based on the demographics of diabetes, but it could be interpreted as racially biased and ignorant of the body composition of people from different ethnic backgrounds. This can affect the applicability of the BMI reading.

Understanding the theory: integrated care boards

If an ICB has a high percentage of Asian residents such as, for example, the West Midlands, then there is likely to be a high incidence of type II diabetes. Therefore, the ICB should ensure that there are enough routing diagnostic tests being done and a high amount of community support for these people. Conversely, just because an area has a low percentage of Asian residents does not mean that they have no residents of an Asian background, so services still need to be designed to meet the needs of all of the population, even if it is a relatively small number of people.

Sickle cell disease

Sickle cell disease is a lifelong blood inherited condition that causes anaemia and severe pain. Anyone can inherit the disease, but both parents need to have the trait in order to pass it on. It is most prevalent in people who are from African and Caribbean backgrounds. There is a lot of information on this condition on the Sickle Cell Society website, the URL of which is included in the further reading section at the end of this chapter.

Coronary heart disease

Coronary heart disease is 50 per cent higher in first-generation South Asians than in white Europeans. There are different thoughts as to why, but it is linked with other comorbidities like diabetes. There is also a higher prevalence of obesity due to a lower uptake of exercise and an apparent higher consumption of fried food (Ho et al., 2022).

Understanding the theory: applying Census data

According to the 2021 Census, the East of England has an increased percentage of Black people living there who will be more likely to have sickle cell disease or coronary heart disease than their white counterparts. These numbers need to be considered when planning health checks and expected attendants to A & E departments in that area.

Maternal death

In the UK, for every 100,000 women who give birth, eight white women will die either during pregnancy or up to six weeks after giving birth. In that same 100,000, 15 Asian women, and 34 Black women will die. The reason for this significant difference in mortality rates is not really known, though there have been studies into this. The general thought is that women from ethnic minorities are not adequately supported or heard by healthcare services as a result of racial bias and therefore don't trust healthcare providers and don't seek help. By promoting unconscious bias training for all healthcare workers, many Trusts are reporting that this gap is being reduced as more understanding is being developed (GOV.UK, 2021a).

There are many other illnesses that are recognised to have a higher incidence in certain ethnic groups. However, as more people are migrating to different countries and adopting different cultural behaviours, the incidence is reducing for those groups. For example, for coronary heart disease there is less of a difference in second- and third-generation South Asians and their European counterparts. This means that as time goes on there will be less need for specific, targeted cardiac awareness in South Asian people and this will have an impact on the health provisions required.

Activity 4.3   Leadership and management

The ICBs need to decide how to allocate their limited funds for their area. They need to provide the most amount of good for the greatest number of people, but such decisions are difficult to make.

- How do you think bias is managed when decisions are being made?
- What services would you prioritise and why?
- How do your biases impact your decision-making?
- How would your priorities impact your community?

As this activity is a personal reflection, no outline answer is provided at the end of the chapter.

Diversity and the law

It is clear that respecting people's differences is paramount to person-centred care. The protected characteristics are protected for a reason, and you are legally obliged to respect them. However, not all practices are protected under law.

Diversity is protected under the Equality Act of 2010 and all measures should be taken to meet the different requirements. However, the Human Rights Act 1998 makes it clear that everyone has the right to life. There have been cases in the UK where parents have been found guilty of neglect as they have allowed their child to die from something that could be treated (like pneumonia). Instead of accessing medical treatment they have prayed for their child, believing that this would help them. These parents believed that they were doing their best for their child and their right to religion is a protected right. However, the Children's Act of 1989 (updated 2004) stipulates that if a child is at risk of harm, then they need to be protected. In these situations, the child becomes a ward of the court and decisions will be made in their best interests without the parents' consent. This is one example of when the law can override a religious belief. This will be explored further in Chapter 8.

Language

The use of appropriate language is a core element of diversity. Now, as one generation succeeds another, certain words that were commonly used have become taboo as it is understood that they are derogatory and offensive. While I shall not list them in this book, I am sure you can think of words which were once used regularly and are now banned from use. It is important that you as a nursing associate make sure that you are using the most up-to-date and correct terminology for the people in your care. One example of a change in language is the use of pronouns. There are many people in society who do not want to be referred to with a gender-specific pronoun and prefer gender-neutral pronouns such as 'them' or 'they'.

Defining terms for ethnicity

There are certain abbreviations which you may have heard such as BME and BAME. BME stands for Black and minority ethnic and BAME stands for Black, Asian and minority ethnic groups and for many years these terms were used to differentiate people with white skin from people without. The two categories (BAME and white) were used as the two defining titles. What this term did was ignore the fact that in a country like England a person could be white but be an immigrant, have English as their second or third language and have a non-English culture. These white people were not recognised in the BAME category as the terminology was too exclusive, which meant that their needs were not being recognised and therefore not being met. It also highlighted some ethnic minority groups over others.

In 2022, through a paper called 'Inclusive Britain', the UK government stopped using the term BAME, instead using terms such as 'ethnic minorities' or 'people from ethnic minority backgrounds'. In Britain, the term ethnic minority means all groups who are not white British (GOV.UK, 2021b).

Chapter summary

This chapter has explored the subject of diversity in the UK. It used the UK Census to identify how different areas within the UK have different diversity needs. It went on to consider some ethnic-specific conditions and the potential impact of this on the NHS.

Useful websites

www.ons.gov.uk/census

The Office of National Statistics is run by the UK government, and its website has all the national statistics you will ever need. It is kept up to date and the data from the Census is interpreted there.

www.nomisweb.co.uk/sources/census_2021

Take some time to look into the diversity in your own neighbourhood using this website.

www.e-lfh.org.uk/programmes/cultural-competence/

NHS England has a cultural competence e-learning package.

www.sicklecellsociety.org/about-sickle-cell/

Learn more about sickle cell from the Sickle Cell Society website.

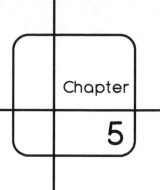

Exploring inclusion

> # Chapter aims
>
> After reading this chapter, you will be able to:
>
> - demonstrate an understanding of some of the health issues faced by some minority groups in the UK;
> - understand good practice used in the NHS to promote inclusivity in healthcare;
> - consider changes that could be incorporated into everyday practice to promote inclusivity.

'Diversity is being invited to the party; inclusion is being asked to dance.' (Verna Myers, 2016)

Introduction

The first pillar of the Code (NMC, 2018a) is 'prioritise people' and the points within that section relate to promoting inclusivity in healthcare. As discussed in other chapters, the UK is a diverse country and the users of the NHS come from a variety of backgrounds and cultures. It is therefore essential that nursing associates understand and respect every person in their care.

This chapter explores the healthcare needs for certain marginalised groups in the UK and offers some suggestions for how to improve inclusivity in healthcare provision. We will also look at marginalised groups in more detail in Chapter 6.

We will begin with a case study from 1998 which considers the challenge of protecting rights of different groups of people who believe in different things.

Case study: *Lee* v *Ashers Baking Company Ltd and others*

In *Lee* v *Ashers Baking Company Ltd and others* (1998) a man asked a bakery in Northern Ireland to bake a cake and decorate it with the words 'support gay marriage'. At this time gay marriage was not legal in Northern Ireland. The bakers refused to do this on religious grounds. It wasn't that they wouldn't bake for a gay man, it was that they felt that they couldn't ice the cake in that way due to their religious beliefs. Mr Lee sued the bakers for discrimination and eventually it was decided that the bakers were not discriminating against Mr Lee. They were maintaining their right to freedom of thought, conscience and religion in accordance with the Human Rights Act 1998.

Activity 5.1   Critical thinking

Consider the Mr Lee case.

- Do you think the right decision was made?

Both sexuality and religion are protected characteristics of the Equality Act.

- Whose rights are more important and why?
- What makes you feel the way that you do?

An outline answer is provided at the end of this chapter.

Department of Health status regarding inclusivity

In 2015 the Department of Health published a framework of guidance for all health professionals to tackle inequalities in healthcare. It was called 'All Our Health: personalised care and population health' (GOV.UK, 2015). The framework aims to protect health, prevent illness and promote wellbeing. It is regularly updated with relevant information as the UK population changes. In 2021, updated specific guidance was published by the Department of Health to help healthcare professionals apply 'All Our Health' in an inclusive manner. In this guidance, the term 'inclusivity' is used to describe those who are socially excluded for any number of reasons, and it highlights that these people will often have multiple risk factors for ill health. They often experience stigma and discrimination and sometimes they aren't in the healthcare system at all. These factors can lead to a lack of access to healthcare and therefore poor health outcomes and large social inequalities. Inclusivity in healthcare, according to this guidance, includes all groups that are socially excluded. A non-exhaustive list includes homeless people, drug and alcohol dependent people, migrant people, sex workers, victims of modern slavery, ex-prisoners and people from Traveller communities. Within each group, needs must be considered on an individual level as we must remember to not dehumanise a group of people with generalisations. This chapter will consider the challenges that some of these excluded groups may face.

Healthcare from the NHS is free for all at the point of delivery. For people in socially excluded groups, it is accessing the service that seems to be the barrier. This could be due to any number of reasons, including being digitally poor, previous bad experiences, language barriers, a fear of being judged or due to something else. If a person doesn't access healthcare early in their journey, then that person may present in A & E when in an acutely unwell state. The 2023 Primary Care Plan aims to improve this by allowing common prescriptions to be available from a pharmacist instead of having to go to a GP. This change should help people access healthcare more easily (NHS England, 2023b).

Examples of inclusive healthcare in the NHS

Decision-making

Since 2010 the UK government in its paper 'No health without mental health' has promoted the idea of 'no decision about me without me' (GOV.UK, 2010). This policy was formed to ensure joint decision-making and increased control for patients. One element of this is ensuring that information is given in a format that the person can understand and that all mechanisms are in place to be able to understand the person's needs. Some people need a strong advocate when they are in hospital, and often that will be the nurse or the nursing associate. In accordance with the Mental Capacity Act 2005, it must be assumed that everyone has capacity and should be involved in their decision-making until it is proved otherwise. As a nursing associate you are likely to be with the service user a lot and therefore you are the best-placed person to support and speak up for that person.

Case study: Inclusivity in a GP practice

You are working in a GP practice and a man in his twenties comes into reception. The policy of the practice is that all appointments must be booked online. He has not booked an appointment as he does not understand the system of how to book an appointment. He may not be registered with your practice; this is unclear. He looks unkempt and has an unpleasant odour. He tells you, in broken English, that he has pain while passing urine and you notice that he has a strong accent, but you do not know where he is from.

Activity 5.2   Decision-making

This young man could be homeless. He could be a sex worker. He could be a migrant, a refugee or an asylum seeker. He could be an ex-convict. He could be none of these things. You do not know anything about him at this time.

How would you, as a nursing associate, support him?
An outline answer is provided at the end of the chapter.

Homelessness

A person is homeless if they do not have a home. This does not mean a person is only homeless if they live on the streets. They are also homeless if they are sofa-surfing, staying in a hostel or squatting. A person is also considered homeless if their home is not a safe place due to poor living conditions or violence, and this is discussed further by the charity Shelter, whose website is included in the further reading section at the end of this chapter.

In 2019 the NHS provided funding for seven specific areas in the UK to support homeless people and their mental health in those areas. This funding was not to solve homelessness, but to ensure that there was support and access to healthcare services for homeless people as and when it was needed. Some areas have specific teams who focus on healthcare for homeless people. For example, in London there is a team that will provide primary healthcare in non-NHS settings. The healthcare team will see people on the street, in day centres or drop-in centres, in hostels and in accessible GP surgeries and provide various different interventions. There are also specialist podiatry and dental services. To provide healthcare to homeless people where they are living means this group can access the support that they need. As a nursing associate it is important to be able to talk with your service users and to allow them to talk to you. To give people the time to trust you and explain their challenges is essential to be able to then offer them support.

Sex workers

Sex workers in the UK are at a high risk of experiencing violence, of drug or alcohol misuse, and of contracting sexually transmitted infections. Unfortunately, sex workers are often reluctant to access healthcare services due to fears of being judged and experiencing prejudice. This fear is recognised within the NHS and while most NHS Trusts do have a free and fully confidential sexual health clinic, some have specific clinics for sex workers in order to respect their privacy and dignity. Many Trusts provide community outreach for those in the sex industry and will visit people in their places of work to offer advice, infectious disease testing, lubricants, condoms and various other items to help maintain their safety. Support is provided to all sex workers irrespective of their background and the type of work that they are in. Counselling as well as physical health support is offered due to the likelihood of trauma and mental health issues being experienced. It is noted by Potter et al. (2022) that these clinics focus on sexual health despite the fact that street sex workers also have a high incidence of chronic diseases. Nonsexual health needs can be missed in sex workers, and they often have a high incidence of poor mental health, including depression, anxiety, post-traumatic stress disorder, self-harm and suicide. Unfortunately, due to the high incidence of substance use disorders in sex workers, they often don't meet the criteria for mental health support services.

As a nursing associate it is important to remember that holistic, person-centred care considers all the needs of the service user, and they must be assessed appropriately.

Migrants

A migrant is a person who has left their home area willingly, usually for economic reasons. This can be nationally or internationally, but it is categorised as a temporary movement as opposed to an immigrant who moves to another country as a permanent resident.

In the case of primary care (GPs and community services) all treatment is free as a temporary patient. Temporary is defined as anything between 24 hours and three months. For secondary services (hospitals and clinics) a person must be an 'ordinary resident'. To be an ordinary resident the status required is 'indefinite leave to remain' but there are exceptions. These exceptions are: care that requires emergency service, end-of-life care, treatment for violence and torture, and the diagnosis and treatment of communicable diseases, Covid-19 and sexually transmitted infections. Refugees, asylum seekers, detainees and victims of trafficking and modern slavery are also entitled to free treatment. As a nursing associate it is not appropriate for you to enquire about someone's residency status. You administer the best care that you can to everyone in your care.

Refugees and asylum seekers

A refugee is a person who has suddenly been forced to leave their home due to violence or war and they are not able to return to their home. They have usually been given refugee status in advance and know that they will have protection when they arrive in a new country.

An asylum seeker has also fled their home country due to danger but they do not have refugee status so they are fleeing without assurance that they will be accepted as a refugee and given protection.

Refugees and asylum seekers have a high incidence of anxiety and post-traumatic stress disorder. They often have physical needs following war and torture. They can struggle to build their lives in the UK.

As a nursing associate you need to consider the person in front of you in a holistic manner and provide the care that they need, allowing time and space for them to express their diverse needs.

Modern slavery and people trafficking

Modern slavery, which as a term includes human trafficking, is a global issue. The UK has a Modern Slavery Act which came into force in 2015 to punish perpetrators and protect victims. People who have been enslaved or trafficked are a high priority for the healthcare services, as victims of modern slavery have very poor physical and mental health. They have been subjected to demanding physical challenges for prolonged periods of time which can lead to physical injury. Those who are sexually exploited also have a high incidence of sexually transmitted infections and post-traumatic stress disorder. Anyone who has been trafficked, exploited or held captive is entitled to free healthcare. However, it can be challenging for this group of people to access healthcare services. When they do present to an NHS provider, they are unlikely to be known to any other services and therefore safely identifying them as vulnerable is essential. Such et al. (2018) discuss the importance of training healthcare workers to be able to identify and support these victims as they are the people likely to meet them at a crisis point. As a nursing associate you may spend a lot of time with these patients and you need to maintain your knowledge and skills to be able to communicate with these vulnerable people.

Prisoners

People detained in a UK prison have full access to the same treatment as anyone else. However, there is prejudice towards people in prison according to a survey published in 2022 by YouGov, which stated that 65 per cent of respondents felt that prison sentences were not harsh enough. Of the people surveyed, many felt that prisoners leave prison with greater access to criminal groups than before they were sentenced and therefore continue to commit crimes once released. The purpose of prison is to help people to rehabilitate and, where possible, rejoin society. For some prisoners, rehabilitation is not possible, but for many it is.

To get paid work once coming out of prison can be challenging and not everyone in this group is able to rejoin society properly. There are big companies in the UK which have a good record of employing ex-offenders. The Timpson Group, for example, is well known for promoting equal opportunity in its employment policy. It employs a high percentage of ex-prisoners and other minority groups. The reasons for this are numerous and include increasing the diversity of the workforce, improving rehabilitation rates for ex-offenders, and promoting the company's public relations.

However, only 17 per cent of ex-offenders get a job within one year of being released (GOV. UK, 2020a). If an ex-offender cannot get a job upon release, maintaining good health can become a challenge and it is easy to fall into a poor health cycle, especially when it is difficult to ensure a stable housing situation without work. As a nursing associate you can work closely with ex-offenders to help them understand how to access support.

Case study: Henry

Henry is working as a nursing associate on a urology ward. A prisoner comes into Henry's ward for treatment. They are accompanied by prison staff, and Henry is told that security for the patient will be provided by the prison staff only. It is made clear that the healthcare team should not supervise the patient alone. The prison staff are scheduled in pairs to cover supervising the patient while they are receiving treatment.

On the patient's third day on the ward one of the prison staff team does not come in due to sickness. Their cover will take about three hours to arrive. Before the second officer arrives, the first officer needs the toilet and Henry is asked, as a nursing associate, to supervise the patient. As soon as Henry is alone with the patient they start to talk to him, asking him a lot of personal questions. They also start to tell him about their history and they ask if Henry wants to know why they are in prison.

Activity 5.3   Critical thinking

Consider the above case study.

- What mistakes have been made in this situation?
- What actions should Henry take at this point?
- What steps could have been taken to not leave the nursing associate alone with the patient?
- How might finding out about the crime affect the ethical principle of justice?
- Can you think of any convictions that might impact on the quality of the care that you deliver?

An outline answer is provided at the end of the chapter.

Travellers

For the first time in 2011, the Census included Gypsies and Travellers as being of 'white other' ethnicity. In 2021 the Roma community was included. This was a big step in inclusivity for this ethnic group, but it has taken a long time considering that they were first categorised as an ethnic minority group in 1976.

It should be noted that not all people in this ethnic group do actually travel. Many live in permanent housing and have done so for at least one generation, but they still consider themselves part of their ethnic and cultural community. In the Census, the Traveller and Roma communities reported low health outcomes in comparison to equivalent categories in the general population. People in this ethnic group are consistently reported as being of lower general health than their equivalents, and the mortality rate for those in the Gypsy and Traveller communities is higher than the rest of the population. In 2016 a report was produced by the Traveller Movement to document the impact on healthcare of the Gypsy and Traveller communities (Greenfields and Brindley, 2016). The study showed that 70 per cent of the people involved in the report lived within 25 miles of where they were born. They were still part of a strong, historic family but, unfortunately, they often experienced racism, and this had led to high levels of negative health in the forms of anxiety and depression. There was also a high incidence of long-term physical illnesses due to a lack of accessing healthcare services. In every healthcare category on the Census, this ethnic group had a high incidence of poor health. The report felt that this was due to the exclusion from society that this ethnic group experiences and poor accommodation standards.

For those living in unauthorised locations, the stress and fear of being moved on from their sites at any time of the day or night also contributed to this poor health. Living with this anxiety and the trauma of being moved on leads to a lot of mental health diagnoses. It also means that there is a lack of continuity of care, lack of follow-up and no therapeutic relationships can be formed with healthcare professionals. People from the Gypsy, Roma and Traveller community are entitled to free NHS healthcare. They can register with a local GP and access healthcare. Unfortunately, there is still a feeling of misunderstanding between the community and the healthcare workers, which still makes them feel isolated and unsupported, meaning that many Traveller communities do not access their GP or local healthcare providers and instead manage their healthcare within their community.

In 2019 a strategy was published to tackle the healthcare inequality faced by this ethnic group and six projects were set up around the country. The sum of £200,000 was devoted to these projects which focus on improving the outcomes of education, social integration and health. Twenty-two further projects have been funded around the country to support Roma communities plus two projects to support the reporting of hate crimes against this minority group (GOV.UK, 2019). These projects are important for providing support for the Traveller community.

As a nursing associate it is important to remember that people from the Traveller community have often had negative experiences with healthcare services so treating without prejudice is essential for this group of people.

Lesbian, gay, bisexual, transgender, queer, intersex, asexual+ (LGBTQIA+)

As you have seen in Chapter 2, the Equality Act of 2010 states that sexual orientation and gender reassignment are protected characteristics. In the NHS, as well as protecting the patients, members of staff also need to be protected. Many members of staff in all healthcare environments are LGBTQIA+ and are often subjected to bullying and harassment from their colleagues. In 2017, Stonewall, a UK-based organisation that fights for the rights of LGBTQIA+ people everywhere, worked with the UK government on a survey focused on the experiences of LGBTQIA+ people in the UK. From the survey, 40 per cent reported experiencing verbal harassment or physical violence due to their sexuality, while 41 per cent felt that healthcare staff lacked understanding of the specific needs of this group of patients (Government Equalities Office, 2018). Some respondents also complained about the number of times they had to explain that they were transgender, or that their partner was the same gender as them. The lack of general understanding and discretion shown to this group of people from NHS workers was a frequent complaint.

As a nursing associate you need to ensure you have a good understanding of the needs of people from this community in order to provide the support that they require. The other major issue identified in this survey was the lack of centres and surgeons who offer transgender treatment in the UK. This leads to long waiting lists, and this has an impact on mental health which then leads to further complications for this group of marginalised people.

As a nursing associate you can work closely with your patients and develop good relationships that enable open communication.

People with a disability

The challenge when working with someone with a disability is to see the person and not the disability, and that is something that you can and must do. Reasonable adjustments need to be made to provide equity for people with a disability, including both patients and staff members. Accessing healthcare can be challenging on a practical level as some NHS hospitals and community centres were built a long time ago and they aren't easy to adjust to suit the needs of a disabled person. All efforts must be made to promote their right to work or to attend appointments and a person with a disability must be supported. As a nursing associate you are the voice of the patients and must embrace that responsibility when promoting their needs.

Minority ethnic groups

According to the 2011 Census, approximately 14 per cent of the UK's population identified as Asian, Black, mixed, or belonging to another ethnic group, while the 2021 Census revealed an increase in that number to approximately 18 per cent. Meanwhile, in 2020 a paper released by the NHS stated that approximately 20 per cent of its workforce was drawn from non-white, ethnic minority groups (GOV.UK, 2020b). A survey taken in 2018 showed that 40 per cent of nurses from an ethnic minority background had experienced bullying, abuse and harassment from patients or members of the public, and 14.5 per cent had experienced discrimination from their colleagues (NHS Providers, 2020). Discrimination in any form from anyone is unacceptable and for it to be so common is a disturbing thought. As a nursing associate, your Code (NMC, 2018a), the values of your Trust and the British values that you work under insist that you treat people fairly and work in an anti-discriminatory manner. But there is discrimination everywhere so you need to be a good role model and highlight when someone else is being discriminatory.

Activity 5.4　　Reflection

Can you think of any situations where a member of staff (or yourself) was affected by bullying, abuse and harassment while at work?

Consider:

- What form did it take (verbal or physical)?
- Was it directed at the person affected, or done behind their back?
- How did that make the person feel?
- Were any actions taken by management?
- If actions were taken, was the victim left satisfied?

As this activity is a personal reflection, no outline answer is provided at the end of the chapter.

People from certain ethnic minority groups have specific healthcare risks and they also have some specific prejudices held against them. Due to this, there has been a push to improve understanding of certain illnesses and how they present, for example sickle cell disease. Patients living with sickle cell disease often report a lack of treatment delivery as they need certain strong painkillers such as opioids. A research document published in 2017 by the National Heart, Lung and Blood Institute (NHLBI) stated that some clinicians seem unwilling to prescribe these painkillers due to fear of addiction when there is no evidence to support the idea that people with sickle cell disease have higher levels of opioid addiction than any other group in society (NHLBI, 2017). This document states that the fear of people with sickle cell disease seeking opioids due to addiction is part of the endemic racism towards people of Black origin. They are often stigmatised as seeking drugs under false pretences and therefore denied the one treatment that works for their pain. This is one example of racism towards patients within healthcare. As a nursing associate it is important to assess each and every patient and not make assumptions based on prejudice.

Covid-19

Covid-19 hit the UK in March 2020. Approximately 73,766 people died in the UK from this respiratory disease in that year alone (ONS, 2020). The statistics on the cases of Covid and the deaths from Covid highlighted the number of vulnerable people in society in the UK. Platt (2021) explored the fact that people from ethnic minorities had a much higher death rate than their white counterparts. Razaq et al. (2020) investigated inequalities in Covid deaths and discovered that although the Black ethnic group makes up 3.5 per cent of the population of England they made up 5.8 per cent of deaths from Covid-19. The figures for Asian ethnicities were similar. Both articles stated that this was due to multiple reasons, including socio-economic status and the types of jobs people from these ethnicities tend to have, living in overcrowded accommodation and ethnicity-related long-term conditions. Once these inequalities were recognised, it became easier to prioritise these groups for vaccines to try to reduce further deaths. This is an example of inclusive healthcare provision, although other questions have been asked about how people from ethnic minorities were treated during the pandemic and this is still being investigated.

Activity 5.5   Reflection

- Can you think of any patients who were overlooked due to their ethnicity? This could be due to a language barrier that was not managed well so their communication was not heard.
- Have you seen a patient deteriorating but it wasn't noticed due to the colour of their skin? A lot of assessments are based on skin colour, but with a patient who is darker skinned, this can be missed by the assessing nurse and nursing associate.
- Have you seen any other treatment issues based on the colour of the patient?

As this activity is a personal reflection, no outline answer is provided at the end of the chapter.

Disabled people working in the NHS

The NHS has over 1.27 million full-time equivalent people working for it (DHSC Media Centre, 2023). It is wise to assume that among that number there will be people living with a disability. Employing someone with a disability requires the employer to make adjustments and these will be explored here.

Activity 5.6   Reflection

The NHS has a legal duty to employ people without prejudice against the protected characteristics of the Equality Act 2010. Thinking about where you have worked within the NHS, consider the following questions:

- How many employees with a physical disability did you see?
- How well equipped was the area for someone with a disability?
- Was there access to all areas if someone were a wheelchair user?
- Was there blue badge parking available for staff?
- In case of an emergency, how would a person in a wheelchair exit the building?

As this activity is a personal reflection, no outline answer is provided at the end of the chapter.

There are some conditions that might prohibit the ability of someone to practise as a nursing associate but only if there is a risk of harm to patients. This would be assessed on a case-by-case basis, and it may be that there are certain areas a person with a disability cannot work in, but they can work in other areas. Somebody's physical ability should not determine whether they can be given a job or not, but there is a risk that people with a disability might not be offered a job due to the unconscious bias of the interviewer. This was discussed in Chapter 3. This risk must be minimised to ensure fairness in the interview process. Good practice must be promoted to minimise discrimination and there are ways to help this, including having more than one person shortlisting and more than one person making the decision of who to hire. Transparency is important and honest reflection of the outcome for each applicant will help to promote justice.

Activity 5.7   Critical thinking

Consider the reasonable adjustments that would need to be made to facilitate a disabled person's right to work in the industry that they have chosen.

- Are there disabilities that you think make healthcare work unachievable?
- Could someone be a nursing associate if they lived with any of the following conditions?

  o   The candidate is wheelchair dependent.
  o   The candidate can mobilise using aids.
  o   The candidate is deaf and requires a signer.
  o   The candidate is blind.
  o   The candidate has a learning difficulty.
  o   The candidate has a chronic or episodic condition like multiple sclerosis or chronic fatigue syndrome.
  o   The candidate has anxiety at times.

Some examples of reasonable adjustments are provided at the end of this chapter.

Activity 5.8   Reflection

Consider healthcare environments you have been in recently as a student, as a member of staff, as a patient or as a visitor, and consider how inclusive each area is.

Physical considerations:

- Were the doorways wide enough for mobility aids?
- Were they automatic doors or did people need to physically open them?
- Were there enough seats for everyone there?
- Were the seats accessible or were they in rows?
- Did the chairs have arms to aid people to lower and rise?
- Was there a lift nearby which was in working order? Were there enough lifts?
- If it was an inpatient facility, was there enough room for wheelchairs in the bedrooms? By the beds? In the bathrooms?

(Continued)

(Continued)

In some older buildings it can be challenging to provide disability access to every area and these shortcomings need to be considered when planning care. If, for example, the building does not have a lift then it is not suitable to put a wheelchair-dependent patient anywhere but the ground floor.

Sensory considerations:

- If patients needed to be called in, was their name called out? Was it easy to hear?
- Did their name flash up on a board? How would blind people know?
- Were signs in large, clear writing for someone with a sight impairment?
- Was there a hearing aid loop available?

Language considerations:

- What language were signs and posters in?
- Were there any translated signs and, if so, into what languages?
- For medical discussions, were translators always present? Were they ever not present? Or were members of the family used? Was that appropriate?
- If information leaflets were available or given to patients, were they available in different languages? Were they offered in different languages to the patients? Was braille offered? Were these choices easily available?

LGBTQIA+ considerations:

- Looking around the wider healthcare area, how many posters or leaflets showed a traditional family? Was there any representation of a non-traditional family structure?
- Are there any gender-neutral toilets available?

Carer considerations:

- Did the environment have enough room for people and their carers?
- Were there enough chairs readily available? If not, was it portrayed as a chore to get more chairs?
- Were there rules on how many people could be in the environment at any one time?
- Did carers and relatives feel welcomed?

Thinking back now, do you think that the environment/s you were thinking of were inclusive?

What changes could be made to increase the inclusivity?
As this is a personal reflection, no answer is offered at the end of this chapter.

Chapter summary

This chapter has considered some marginalised groups of people who live, work and access healthcare in the UK. It has identified some specific needs for these groups and highlighted good practice within the NHS that promotes inclusivity. It also considered where improvements could be made and how a nursing associate could be involved in these changes.

Activities: Brief outline answers

Activity 5.1

You probably feel instinctively that the judge was either right or wrong in their ruling. It would be helpful to explore why you felt that way. It may be due to personal reasons like your own religious beliefs or your own sexuality. However, when considering inclusivity, everyone must be included. No one's rights should be considered to be more important than anyone else's. At the time of this case, gay marriage was not legal in Northern Ireland, which could support the religious standpoint slightly more. Alternatively, you could argue that the gay community was more oppressed in Northern Ireland at that time so needed more support. There is justification for either judgement.

Activity 5.2

- This man needs to be seen then and there and not be sent away to book an appointment online despite the fact that it is the policy of the practice.
- He may need to be helped to register with the practice.
- An interpreter may need to be sourced to support him during appointments.
- Gentle, open communication methods will need to be used to try to get a comprehensive patient assessment.
- Knowledge of local services available to him is essential.
- Follow-up appointments may need to be made for him so he has support and a contact.

Activity 5.3

- It is imperative that Henry remains professional with all patients at all times. The reason healthcare staff shouldn't know about the crime of prisoners is because it can have an impact on the care delivered, which then puts you, the nurse associate, at risk of negligence. There are certain convictions that may impact the care that you are delivering.
- Henry should not have been left alone with that patient as that is against policy. Another member of the nursing team should have been with Henry to ensure that he was not alone.
- The prison officer needed to be able to go to the toilet so steps should have been taken to ensure that Henry was not on his own.
- All patients are entitled to the best care possible and their social history must not impact upon that.

Activity 5.7

The candidate is wheelchair dependent.

A wheelchair user would need to work in an area with enough space to move the wheelchair. A desk may need to be lowered to ensure they can reach the computer. A hands-on caring role might be challenging for a wheelchair-dependent person, but there are other roles and areas within healthcare that could be taken.

The candidate can mobilise using aids.

An allowance for extra rest may be required for this person. A hands-on caring role may be possible depending on the specific needs of the person, but the type of care involved may need to be considered.

The candidate has a hearing impairment and requires a sign language interpreter.

Permission would need to be sought from all service users and families to have an extra person present for intimate care, but working as a nursing associate is possible. Ensuring hearing loops and deaf-friendly software is available may be helpful depending on the impairment.

The candidate has a sight impairment.

There are different degrees of sight impairment so each person would need to be considered on a case-by-case basis. If the person has some vision then adjustments can be made, for example providing documents in large text and providing colour filters where appropriate. If someone is completely blind then working as a nursing associate may not be possible. However, working in the NHS is still possible for a blind person once reasonable adjustments have been made.

The candidate has a learning difficulty.

The degree of the learning difficulty may affect the person's ability to work as a nursing associate, but a career in the NHS is still possible for anyone with a learning difficulty. The person would need to be assessed in order to ensure the role is appropriate.

If the candidate has a chronic or episodic condition like multiple sclerosis or chronic fatigue syndrome, an awareness of the condition would be required by everyone who worked with that person, but a career as a nursing associate is definitely possible. Adjustments would need to be made to allow for appropriate rest and recuperation and the shift pattern that they work.

The candidate has anxiety.

Awareness and understanding of the individual needs of a person with anxiety issues would be required by everyone working with them, so the symptoms could be managed when needed. A career as a nursing associate is possible for someone with anxiety when the person is understood and adjustments are made.

Useful websites

www.stonewall.org.uk

Stonewall is a charity dedicated to promoting the rights of everyone in the LGBTQIA+ community. It keeps its website up to date with opinion pieces and news reports and provides a voice for people who sometimes cannot speak for themselves.

www.ons.gov.uk

The Office of National Statistics is run by the UK government, and its website has all the national statistics you will ever need. It is kept up to date and the data from the Census is interpreted there.

https://england.shelter.org.uk/

Shelter is a UK charity which campaigns for housing for everyone.

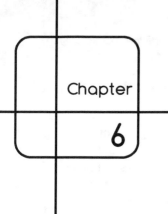

Exploring equity and equality

NMC STANDARDS OF PROFICIENCY FOR NURSING ASSOCIATES

This chapter will address the following platforms and proficiencies:

Platform 1: Being an accountable professional

1.1   understand and act in accordance with the Code: Professional standards of practice and behaviour for nurses, midwives and nursing associates, and fulfil all registration requirements

1.5   understand the demands of professional practice and demonstrate how to recognise signs of vulnerability in themselves or their colleagues and the action required to minimise risks to health

1.11   provide, promote, and where appropriate advocate for, non-discriminatory, person-centred and sensitive care at all times. Reflect on people's values and beliefs, diverse backgrounds, cultural characteristics, language requirements, needs and preferences, taking account of any need for adjustments

Platform 2 : Promoting health and preventing ill health

2.4   understand the factors that may lead to inequalities in health outcomes

Chapter aims

After reading this chapter, you will be able to:

- understand the difference between equality and equity;
- consider the protected characteristics of the Equality Act and the impact that they have on your practice;
- understand how discrimination can lead to oppression;
- explore the principle of justice and how to apply that to everyday practice.

'All animals are equal, but some animals are more equal than others.' (George Orwell, 1949)

Introduction

This epigraph above is a famous quote from a novel first published in 1949 and is just as true today as it was then. The NHS is free for all at the point of delivery, but for reasons we will look at, it is not accessible to all. This chapter will look at the definitions of equality, equity, discrimination and oppression and will then work through the nine protected characteristics of the Equality Act 2010, considering how different groups are marginalised and oppressed. The chapter will consider the role of the nursing associate when supporting these groups of people.

Equality and healthcare provision

In healthcare it is essential that people have what is considered 'fair treatment', and equality is intrinsically linked with the ethical principle of justice. However, there are different thoughts as to how that can be managed. As seen in Chapter 1, Beauchamp and Childress (2019) consider the principle of justice and healthcare allocation from different perspectives. They consider whether resources should be allocated according to need, or by equal share, or for other reasons like the patient being an army veteran or someone who has paid taxes all their life. All of these could be considered justifiable ways to allocate resources on a day-to-day basis.

When considering healthcare provision on a bigger scale, the NHS needs to look beyond the individual. The NHS Constitution states that the *NHS is committed to providing best value for taxpayers money and the most effective, fair and sustainable use of finite resources* (GOV.UK, 2023a). Therefore, it is impossible to look at each individual story. Allocation of funds must be based on a consequentialist perspective: in other words, what will do the most amount of good for the greatest number of people. For example, after research trials on a new medication or treatment are evaluated, the option which is the most cost effective is chosen in order to offer it to as many people as possible. That may mean that every person who is diagnosed with a certain illness is offered the same treatment. However, that may mean that some people don't get the exact medication that they need, but it also means that more people can get some form of treatment. This is treating everyone the same and practising equality. Equity, however, is different.

Equity and healthcare provision

Equity can be considered a fairer form of equality. It is different from equality as it focuses on the individual and it is the very essence of person-centred care. It does not assume that everybody with the same diagnosis has the exact same clinical needs, but instead it tailors treatment to the individual person. This is not practicable on a national level, but on an everyday allocation of your care, it is. You, as a nursing associate, need to look at each patient you are caring for and meet their individual needs. You cannot give the same care to every patient as each patient has their own needs which you must care for.

Every person under the care of the NHS should have fair care and fair treatment at all times including the care they receive from their nursing associate. Unfortunately, there are times where people are not treated fairly and are discriminated against. This will be explored here.

Discrimination

There are multiple forms of discrimination that people are exposed to every day (see Table 6.1). To discriminate is not always a negative process – it is to note a difference. Issues arise when people are treated in a certain way due to the noted difference. This is normally considered to be a negative, but there can be cases of positive discrimination. The focus of this chapter is negative discrimination.

Table 6.1 Types of discrimination

Stereotyping	The same assumptions are made about a group of people, about their characters, behaviours and needs, with no consideration of the individuals in that group.
Marginalisation	Certain groups of people are pushed to the outskirts of society and therefore have restricted access to available services.
Invisibilisation	The process of certain groups not being seen in favour of other, more powerful groups.
Welfarism	The assumption that certain groups of people require certain interventions without considering any individual factors.
Infantilisation	The process of demeaning adults by talking to them or about them as if they were children. For example, calling women 'girls' or men 'boys' or using childlike language with an adult.
Medicalisation	The situation where someone is given the title of being ill and therefore that becomes their main identifying factor.
Dehumanisation	The process of giving groups of people titles which take away their human aspects. For example, 'the elderly' or 'generation X' or 'the disabled'.
Trivialisation	The process of undermining discriminatory practice by making it seem insignificant or minor; not a major issue that needs consideration.

There are occasions where a person is subjected to multiple different types of discrimination. For example, a person over the age of 80 may be stereotyped as being elderly and therefore dehumanised, spoken down to, medicalised as having common, age-related issues and subjected to welfarism by having referrals made that they might not need. Another example is when a person with a learning difficulty is infantilised, stereotyped and dehumanised. They can become invisible while their carer or family member accompanying them is spoken to instead. Also common is when a person living with long-term, life-limiting conditions like motor neurone disease or Parkinson's disease is stereotyped, medicalised and becomes invisible in healthcare situations while their carers are communicated with instead.

Discrimination can arise through a thoughtless opinion that people may not know they have (known as unconscious bias, as discussed in Chapter 3) and they may not have a malicious intention. Intended or not, damage is still caused, and oppression still occurs. Ingrained, unexpected discrimination is dangerous as discrimination in any form leads to the oppression of a certain part of society. Any discrimination to a protected characteristic becomes oppression (Thompson, 2020), and the different forms of oppression will be discussed in this chapter.

The Equality Act 2010

The Equality Act of 2010 was introduced in Chapter 1 and the nine protected characteristics were identified. Each protected characteristic is vulnerable to oppression and abuse, and the different forms of oppression are shown in Table 6.2.

Each form of oppression will be considered here to identify common discrimination that can be seen every day.

Table 6.2 Discrimination and oppression

Categories of discrimination (from the Equality Act 2010)	→	Forms of oppression
Age	→	Ageism
Disability	→	Ableism
Gender reassignment	→	Transgender oppression
Marriage and civil partnership	→	Heterosexism
Pregnancy and maternity	→	Pregnancy discrimination
Race	→	Racism
Religion of belief	→	Religious oppression
Sex	→	Sexism
Sexual orientation	→	Heterosexism

Ageism

Age discrimination is used against younger people and older people at different times. People are too young for senior jobs, or people are too old for active jobs. People of different ages can be infantilised and patronised and their voices are sometimes not heard. They can be medicalised also, and decisions made on their behalf based on their age and their diagnosis, not on the person that they are. When people are referred to as 'the elderly', for example, it dehumanises a large group of people and takes away the principle of person-centred care.

Elder abuse

Age abuse can take many forms: verbal, physical, sexual, psychological, financial, neglectful and more. It can be at an individual level or an institutional level. According to the World Health Organization (WHO, 2022), one in six people over the age of 60 experience elder abuse in the community. In residential and nursing home settings that number increases. It is expected that this number will continue to increase due to a growing elderly population across the world.

Case study: Discharging a patient

You are working on a ward and a man aged 83 is ready to go home following a knee arthroscopy. He is fully mobile and his pain is minimal. He lives alone and has done so since he was 75. The nursing team is concerned about how he will cope at home alone. Your colleagues want an occupational therapist to assess his home before he is discharged, but he is both upset and insulted by this referral and wants to make a complaint about ageism. He feels that they have made this referral based on his age, not his ability.

Activity 6.1   Critical thinking

As a nursing associate, how could you support this man and his successful discharge home?
An outline answer is provided at the end of the chapter.

Presumptions are made about people with certain characteristics. Many people live beyond all expectations, as we can see in Activity 6.2.

Activity 6.2   Reflection

Fauja Singh, born in 1911, took up marathon running in his eighties and ran his final marathon at the age of 101. He is a great example of age being just a number.

Can you think of any activities that age and age alone prevents you from doing?
As this activity is a personal reflection, no outline answer is provided at the end of the chapter.

Ableism

Ableism is discrimination against people with a disability. The noun 'disability' (from the Latin 'lack of' or 'not') is itself discriminatory as it immediately states that certain members of society are not as able as others. They are lacking in an ability that they should have. That language puts them at a disadvantage to others. They are different from the 'normal', making them 'abnormal', and the implication is that they should be helped to be 'normal' again as being 'disabled' is something to avoid as a disabled person must have a poor quality of life.

The following case study is of a woman who is a living illustration of the harm that ableism can cause.

Case study: Baroness Jane Campbell

Jane Campbell was born in 1959 and when she turned one her mother was told she had a diagnosis of spinal muscular atrophy and that she wouldn't reach the age of two. However, she has since gone on to become well educated and holds two degrees. She is a passionate supporter of disability rights and has three honorary degrees. She tells a story of being admitted to hospital in 2010 with a chest infection – bilateral pneumonia. She and her husband were told by a doctor that she was very ill, and that if they put her on a ventilator it would be really difficult to wean her off it. As she wouldn't want to be attached to a ventilator forever, they

(Continued)

simply wouldn't start it. Her husband protested and argued that all interventions should be used to prolong her life. The next day a different doctor was there who said the same thing and wanted to allow her to die. Again, the husband advocated on Jane's behalf, explaining she had everything to live for. He asked them to treat Jane like any woman with pneumonia and look beyond her disability. They changed their perspective and their medical plan and actively saved her life. She is still active in campaigning for disability rights today. Her website gives an interesting perspective of living with a disability and this can be found in the further reading section at the end of this chapter.

Baroness Campbell is an example of someone being medicalised and infantilised without considering her as a person. She was judged by her diagnosis, not by the person. This was not an example of person-centred care.

When people are given a title which automatically invokes an image of that person, presumptions can be made, and prejudice can occur. The previous two case studies are real-life examples which demonstrate why you must keep your mind open, not prejudge your patient and, instead, treat everyone as an individual with specific needs. You also need to consider how you refer to a patient, as language is so important in healthcare. For example, whenever you, as a nursing associate, state that a person 'suffers from' or 'suffers with' you are assuming that their quality of life is diminished because of the long-term condition or disability. People live with their diagnosis; they are not all suffering from it. To assume they are suffering is to medicalise them and dehumanise them.

We explored micro-assaults in Chapter 3 and there are many that promote a lack of equality for someone with a disability. They are prejudicial and damaging but they are used in everyday language by many people.

Activity 6.3 Reflection

Consider the following micro-assaults for disabled people in everyday language:

'Falling on deaf ears'
'Turning a blind eye'
'He is crazy today'
'I'm having a bipolar day'
'That is so lame'
'I'm being dumb today'
'He has a blindspot for her'
'I was paralysed with fear'
'My workload is crippling'
'Her OCD is kicking in about the cleaning'
'The blind leading the blind'

How often do you use these sayings, or similar? How could you word them differently?
An outline answer is provided at the end of this chapter.

Transgender oppression

Gender reassignment is becoming increasingly prevalent and although it might still feel quite new, it has a long history.

- The first transgender female to male surgery in the UK happened between 1946 and 1949 and male to female in 1951. Gender reassignment surgery was not legal at this time, and this was therefore hidden.
- In the 1970s it became legal in the UK to change someone's gender on a passport and driving licence.
- In 1999 the right to access medical treatment for gender reassignment was established.
- In 2002 the Lord Chancellor's Office officially declared that transexuality is not a mental illness, but a recognised medical condition characterised by an overpowering sense of different gender identity.
- In 2004, thanks to the Gender Recognition Act, it became possible for people in the UK to legally change their gender. Reassignment surgery is not a requirement, but the person needs to have lived in their 'new' gender for at least two years.
- In 2010 gender reassignment became a protected characteristic in the Equality Act.
- In 2019 the World Health Organization declassified transgender health issues as a mental health condition.
- In 2022 Dominic Raab stated that prisoners would be sent to prisons based on their genitalia, not based on how they identify.

Case study: Stephanie

Stephanie, a transgender woman, is admitted to your gynaecological ward as her prostate is enlarged. Due to the patient being in a hospital bay, when the doctors review her, it is clear that they are discussing her prostate. Other patients can hear the assessment and understand that Stephanie is transgender. Some of the patients complain about Stephanie being on their ward and would like to be transferred as they feel vulnerable and uncomfortable with her there.

Activity 6.4   Work-based learning

Consider the case study above.

- What can be done to protect everyone in this situation?
- As a nursing associate, what can you do to promote equality and equity?

An outline answer is provided at the end of the chapter.

Heterosexism

Heterosexism can be expressed in multiple ways. One way is where male–female relationships are considered to be 'normal' and any diversion from that 'normal' is 'abnormal'. The Marriage (Same Sex Couples) Act 2013 meant same-sex couples can legally marry, but that does not mean that this is accepted by everyone. There are assumptions that some people make about what is normal and any partnerships that do not conform to these can be discriminated against.

Pregnancy discrimination

For some employers, hiring women who may go on maternity leave seems like a negative move for their company. However, it is against the law to not employ someone because they have children or plan to have children. Women also need to be allowed the time for antenatal care and are entitled to 52 weeks maternity leave. How much the employer pays towards the maternity leave, however, is up to the employer and the contracts and policies of the company. Employers are also required to provide a safe place for breastfeeding or expressing milk postpartum.

Case study: Nadia

Nadia is a staff nurse working in a stroke rehabilitation centre. She is six months pregnant. She is struggling more and more with the heavy nature of the workload and is doing less of the work than expected as it is making her back really painful. She has asked her manager for a lighter workload, but they suggested that she takes sick leave. If she does take sick leave, then her maternity leave would have to start and that would reduce the amount of time she could stay at home once the baby is born. She does not want this, but she is unable to do a lot of the hands-on nursing care now.

The baby is born, and Nadia returns to work once the baby is eight months old. She is still breastfeeding her child and plans to do so for 18 months. She therefore needs to express milk while she is working.

Activity 6.5 Work-based learning

Consider the case study above.

- What should be done to support Nadia?
- What impact would that have on the team?
- What is the responsibility of the line manager here?

An outline answer is provided at the end of the chapter.

Racism

One example of discrimination that relates directly to equality and equity is the use, or lack of use, of translators with patients for whom English is not their first language. Often translators are not used, and family members are relied upon to provide translation (MacLellan et al., 2022), which brings significant issues. In its 'Guidance for commissioners' (2018), NHS England states that every patient has a right to a translator, and it is the responsibility of the care provider to ensure that an appropriately qualified registered interpreter is booked. Using a friend or family member is not considered good practice and is strongly discouraged, and as a nursing associate you need to make sure you advocate for your patients by encouraging the use of translators. Realistically, translators cannot be used all the time, but there are other methods of communication, for example, picture cards with simple everyday topics like a picture of a toilet or some tablets or a glass of water. As a nursing associate you can help ensure these tools are in place.

Activity 6.6   Critical thinking

- Are translators used appropriately in your workplace?
- Does every patient for whom English is not their first language have a translator provided for their care? If not, how is consent to carry out treatment obtained?
- Who is used and are they appropriate?
- Have you ever seen any problems arise by not using official translators?
- What have you seen used when translators are not available?

An outline answer is provided at the end of the chapter.

Microaggressions faced by people with a disability were considered earlier in this chapter. Here are examples of race-based microaggressions. In Chapter 3 we considered the complex issue of unconscious bias and the microaggressions that often come with it. The following reflective exercise asks you to consider your own behaviours.

Activity 6.7   Reflection

Here are some examples of potentially microaggressive racist language:

'So where are you from? /Where are you really from?'
'Is your partner also Indian/Chinese/Italian, etc?'
'I don't think of you as brown/Black/non-white.'
'I don't see colour.'
'What colour is your child?'

Now consider the following:

- Have you ever asked any of those questions?
- Have you ever been asked any of those questions?
- Many people ask these questions and do not know that they are being offensive, a fact which needs to be remembered.

Now that you can recognise these microaggressions, you can challenge people about their language.
   As this activity is a personal reflection, no outline answer is provided at the end of the chapter.

Religious oppression

The right to religion, including to not have a religion, is a right protected by the Equality Act. In healthcare there are many situations where awareness of religious requirements is needed. There are specific rituals that people need to perform, and it is essential that these are respected. There may be specific requirements of Muslim women in maternity care (Firdous et al., 2020), for example, which are completely different to the needs of a Catholic woman or a woman with no religion. That is not to say that you are expected to know all of the requirements of all of the different religions in this country, but the patients should be asked if they have any particular requirements or needs, and you must listen. Different religions have different requirements for prayer time and eating rituals among other things, and these need to be respected, but patient care should still come first. It is important that all members of staff understand the exceptions to religious rituals when patients are involved. There are some well-known religious beliefs that can lead to conflict for all healthcare professionals. For example, a Jehovah's Witness refuses a lifesaving blood transfusion on religious grounds and this refusal leads to their death. This is a challenge for healthcare professionals, but if that is the decision the patient makes then that needs to be accepted.

Religion is often seen as very important in end-of-life care and research has shown that people feel less anxious when their religious needs are met. People, when faced with a difficult decision or situation, will often turn to their religion, so a good understanding of their religion will be helpful.

Equality is applicable to all and someone who holds religious beliefs has as many rights as someone who does not. The following case study from 2013 illustrates a situation where two different parties have diametrically opposing views and there is no compromise that can be made to please both groups.

Case study: Religious symbols

In 2013, staff nurse Shirley Chaplin was instructed to remove her necklace which was a Christian cross. She refused on religious grounds, but the employment tribunal ruled with her employer, and she had to remove the necklace.

In 2020, staff nurse Mary Onuoha was forced out of her job due to wearing a Christian cross on her necklace. In 2022 the employment tribunal concluded that this was a breach of her right to religion and ruled that she could wear it. Physical manifestations like a cross, a hijab, turbans, kalava bracelets and more are now permitted to be worn by healthcare professionals. This debate took a long time to resolve but it does now allow for equality and equity for all religions and for people without religions.

Sexism

Sexism is judging a person based purely on their gender. Sexism can affect anyone, although it is typically thought of as being more applicable to women. There are many forms of sexism, and some seem insignificant compared to others, but they are all forms of oppression.

Hostile sexism versus benevolent sexism (microaggressions) against women

Hostile sexism is where women are considered the inferior sex. It is, for example, when women are seen as being not as strong as men, not as clever as men and not as capable as men. They can be patronised, judged on their looks and overlooked for promotion in preference to their male counterparts (Moffat, 2021). There is also the issue of the gender pay gap – in the NHS there is an acknowledged pay gap between the genders. According to a report published by NHS England in 2021, the mean gender pay gap is an astonishing 8.4 per cent (NHS England, 2021).

Benevolent sexism is also common and not often seen as inappropriate. It is the process of praising women for maintaining the 'traditional' female roles. It is still assumed in society that it is the role of the woman to bring up the children, to look after the home and to take care of people. It is also assumed that men are the main earners in a family. This can often be portrayed in a microaggressive unconscious way. For example, if a child gets their clothes dirty, they are told that their mummy will clean them, with no knowledge of who actually does the clothes cleaning in that child's world. Likewise, stating that women are great at multitasking is another example of benevolent sexism.

Activity 6.8   Critical thinking

- Do you find that in healthcare there is an assumption of who is the nurse and who is the doctor based on their gender?
- On the course you studied to become a nursing associate, what was the gender mix? Were/are there more men or more women on your course, or was/is it about the same? Why do you think that is?

As this activity is a personal reflection, no outline answer is provided at the end of the chapter.

Activity 6.9   Reflection

Can you think of any microaggressions or assumptions that you have witnessed regarding the 'normal' image of a family?

An outline answer is provided at the end of the chapter.

Marginalised groups

There are many groups within society that are discriminated against in a way that leads to them being excluded from access to healthcare. They don't fit into the protected characteristics of the Equality Act and can be neglected by the whole system.

Those without a fixed address

In order to access healthcare in the UK, everyone needs to be registered with a GP. There is an assumption that it is not possible to register with a GP unless you have a fixed address. Homeless people do not have a fixed address; neither do some people from the Traveller, Roma or Gypsy communities; nor do sofa-surfers or some asylum seekers or refugees. If people from these groups do not register with a GP they cannot access any required healthcare interventions. However, the NHS is quite clear that a temporary address can be given, such as a friend's address or a day centre that is within the catchment area of the surgery. If a temporary address is not available, the GP can use the surgery's address as the permanent address. Although such allowances are made, they are not widely known among this vulnerable group and therefore they do not have equal access to healthcare.

'Unhealthy' lifestyle choices

People who have addictions often hesitate before seeking support due to fear of being judged. The prejudice that people exhibit towards an alcoholic, a drug user, a morbidly obese person or a sex worker is often apparent, which makes these vulnerable people avoid getting help. The lack of equality and equity in access then causes a real health risk for these groups of people.

Activity 6.10   Reflection

- Can you think of people who have been treated unfavourably and may have been put off accessing healthcare?
- What could you as a nursing associate have done to help this person?

As this activity is a personal reflection, no outline answer is provided at the end of the chapter.

Chapter summary

This chapter has considered the difference between equity and equality and rationalised why equity is a more suitable goal. It has considered marginalised groups based on the Equality Act of 2010 and the challenges that these groups face. It has also highlighted and further explored the concepts of microaggression and unconscious bias which were introduced in Chapter 3.

Activities: Brief outline answers

Activity 6.1

You need to check that a full assessment has been done on this man. Objective information is key here and should be based on ability not age. There is no reason to assume that the 83-year-old patient cannot take full care of himself, especially as there were no issues before he came in. Person-centred care means the individual must be assessed based on his needs and ability, not his age.

Activity 6.3

Falling on deaf ears	consider	Not receptive to the information
Turning a blind eye	consider	Ignoring the incident right now
He is crazy today	consider	He is not behaving like he usually does today
I'm having a bipolar day	consider	I am not feeling like myself today
That is so lame	consider	I do not like this activity
I'm being dumb today	consider	I am not understanding the task
He has a blind spot for her	consider	He is unable to notice her faults
I was paralysed with fear	consider	I was so scared I couldn't move
My workload is crippling	consider	My workload is rather large right now
Her OCD is kicking in about the cleaning	consider	She is fastidious with cleaning
The blind leading the blind	consider	No one really knows how to do this

Activity 6.4

There is no easy answer to this situation. The patient could be moved to a side room, although that is not a good use of resources. If they don't feel comfortable on a male ward, then it is unfair for them to be sent there. Communication is necessary to try to meet the needs of all the patients, but it is a delicate situation. As a nursing associate you need to take the time to talk to all patients involved and offer support to everyone as no one's needs are more important than someone else's.

Activity 6.5

Your colleague is entitled to work, and her employer should consider the workload and adjust it accordingly in order to reduce the risk to her. If this happens then other members of the team are likely to be given extra duties, which could cause tension, so this would need to be explained to the team.

Employers need to provide space and time for a mother to express her breast milk for as long as she wishes to breastfeed.

Activity 6.6

Are translators used appropriately in your workplace?

This is a personal reflective answer based on your own experiences.

Does every patient for whom English is not their first language have a translator provided for their care? If not, how is consent obtained?

Family members are often relied upon to translate if an official translator has not been arranged. There are also incidents of other members of staff being asked to translate – doctors, nurses, technicians and domestic staff. This means that consent is obtained through assuming that the translation has been done correctly and truthfully with no errors in either direction.

Who is used and are they appropriate?

NHS policies and local guidelines state to only use official translators. The issue of using non-official translators is that they may not know the more technical medical words in the required language. Also, family members may be put in an uncomfortable position if, for example, they need to break bad news. They may not be willing to do that and they shouldn't be asked to. They may not translate correctly, either intentionally or non-intentionally.

Have you ever seen any problems arise by not using official translators?

This is a personal reflective answer based on your own experiences.

What have you seen used when translators are not available?

This is a personal reflective answer based on your own experiences.

Activity 6.9

There are many examples that could be given, these are just two:

Saying 'When is your husband/wife coming?' to a patient without knowing their status.

Or asking a same sex couple 'Which one of you has the mum or dad role?'

Further reading

Historic England (n.d.) Trans pioneers. Available at: **https://historicengland. org.uk/research/inclusive-heritage/lgbtq-heritage-project/trans-and-gender-nonconforming-histories/trans-pioneers**

Read this article to learn more about the history of transgender rights.

Useful websites

https://baronesscampbellofsurbiton.uk

Learn more about Baroness Jane Campbell and her fight for the rights of disabled people.

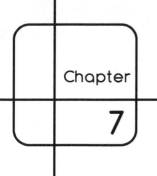

Delivering person-centred care

Chapter aims

After reading this chapter, you will be able to:

- understand the needs of different religions in end-of-life care;
- understand how to provide person-centred end-of-life care;
- explore the holistic assessment of a patient and the EDI factors that impact that;
- consider the importance of effective communication in healthcare.

Understanding the theory: key terminology

Assessment – the process of considering the health of the patient.

Holistic care – looking at the patient not only from a physical perspective, but also considering their psychological and social needs.

Person-centred care – including the patient in all decisions made about them to ensure that their best interests are met.

Introduction

This chapter will consider the task of delivering person-centred care and the way in which EDI relates directly to this.

It will consider specific clinical situations including end-of-life care and the assessment of a patient. The nursing associate role within the multidisciplinary team will be explored, as will the importance of effective communication skills. Scenarios will be used to demonstrate how to apply theory to practice.

The Code

One of the pillars of the Code (NMC, 2018a) is prioritising people. In order to do this, nurses, midwives and nursing associates are told to treat every person as an individual and to ensure that they uphold the dignity of that person. As a nursing associate you must listen to your patients and their relatives and act on their individual needs. You have to look at people holistically and always act in their best interests. You also need to respect their right to privacy and their right to confidentiality while delivering high-quality person-centred care. You have to offer the best care available and sometimes what may be the best medical care is not the care that the patient wants. Respecting the patient's choice when you don't agree with it can be challenging, but the rights of that patient are paramount, as we noted in Chapters 1 and 2.

The role of the nursing associate

The nursing associate role was designed to act as a bridge between the registered nurse and the healthcare assistant. The nursing assistant should be able to identify risks and administer high-level care in a way that the healthcare assistant cannot. The nursing assistant spends time performing clinical tasks with each patient and should therefore be able to get to know each patient and create a rapport with them. This rapport should lead to an understanding of the patient by the nursing assistant, which then enables them to be relied upon to advocate for each of their patients, support their needs and ensure that patient-centred care is maintained. The next section will expand on the theory of person-centred care.

The sick role

In 1951 Talcott Parsons wrote about the 'sick role' (Parsons, 1951). His theory looked only at acute illness, not long-term conditions. The four components of the theory are:

1. The person who is sick is not responsible for being sick.
2. The person who is sick is exempt from certain social requirements while they are sick, like working, for example.
3. As being sick is temporary, the unwell person must try to get better.
4. In order to get better, the sick person must seek and follow medical advice.

Parsons' idea links with the medical theory of healthcare, where the medical team makes decisions for the patients and the patients comply with what they are told to do. Society has developed over the years and while it is expected that medical professionals can offer appropriate treatment, the role of the patient in their care has changed. The patient now sets the goals and priorities, and the healthcare professionals must work with them to find the right treatment. This level of person-centred care is essential to provide fair and equitable care (Coulter and Oldham, 2016).

While healthcare has developed over the past 70 years, the medical model is still very present. People do lose some of their independence when they are not well. An example of this is the wearing of the hospital gown. When a person is admitted to hospital they are often put straight into a hospital gown and this process has an impact on them. Morton et al. (2020) discuss the fact that when a person puts on a gown, they become a patient. By putting on the gown the person gives up their independence and becomes both emotionally and physically vulnerable. The traditional hospital gown also does not allow for some religious requirements for women to remain covered. This is not inclusive practice. In 2006 Lancashire Teaching Hospital introduced an 'interfaith gown' which was designed like a burka but also provided access for healthcare professionals. This style of gown would make Muslim women feel more comfortable in hospital, but it is unclear as to how widely they are used. Respecting the culture of each patient is fundamental to enhance patient care.

Person-centred care

Person-centred care is mentioned a lot in documents written for healthcare professionals. The emphasis on the patient being the centre of the care is reinforced frequently. The policy of *no decision about me without me* (Coulter and Collins, 2011) is an integral part of person-centred care. This policy explains the practice of shared decision-making where all decisions about tests and treatment plans are made based on both evidence-based practice and the patient's preferences once they have been given all the information.

While person-centred care is a cornerstone of healthcare delivery, it is important to remember that the patient still needs to receive medical advice and be given all the information about their condition and treatment options. The person may not want to be given information, or the family might not want them to receive it, but they still must be told even if that seems to override the concept of person-centred care. A decision can only be made if it is informed – and remember (as discussed in Chapter 2) a decision does not need to be wise to be valid.

Every person has a different belief of what quality of life constitutes, of what is appropriate treatment, and of how they want to live their lives. They need to be given time and space to make the decisions that are asked of them. The communication skills required to allow for this are very important and will be explored further here.

Communication skills

Activity 7.1   Critical thinking

Imagine being in a situation where you are somewhere you haven't been before and you are in a room with one person who you have never met before. This stranger starts asking you questions about your bodily functions, your family situation, your physical abilities and your likes and dislikes. The stranger is in quite a rush as they are busy and need you to answer these personal questions quickly.

- How do you feel in this situation?
- How comfortable would you be if you needed to disclose personal information to a stranger?

Now imagine this stranger speaks a different language to you but still asks these personal questions and needs you to answer them quickly.

- How do you feel in this situation?
- How easy would it be to disclose personal information to someone who didn't speak the same language as you?

As this activity is a personal reflection, no outline answer is provided at the end of the chapter.

In healthcare, patients are expected to answer a lot of personal questions in a short space of time. The questions are asked because information is needed in order to provide appropriate care, but for some people it may include information they are not comfortable sharing. Some subjects might be really challenging for the person to discuss, but they are expected to divulge everything multiple times to strangers. This is why effective communication skills are so important.

Annex A of the Standards of Proficiency for Nursing Associates (NMC, 2018b) outlines the communication skills required of you as a nursing associate. Communication is essential in providing effective person-centred care and it is important to remember that listening is an essential part of communication. Patients will give information if they are allowed the time to do so, but there is also a lot to be understood from the silences. Nursing associates need to be able to interpret body language and allow patients time to communicate.

Effective communication is essential for the assessment of a patient. It is often advised that you ask open questions and avoid closed questions (Afriyie, 2020) in order to allow a person to give you information. The importance of providing enough time is often highlighted to encourage someone to communicate with you. Your posture and stance are also important, so sitting down, for example, lets the person feel that you have time for them and that they are important to you. This also helps to develop a relationship of trust which makes assessing them more accurate as they may give you more information.

Many patients do not speak English fluently and use family members to support them at their appointments. The appropriateness of this does need to be considered for each intervention you perform. There are other communication methods that can be useful for patients, for example, picture cards illustrating what the patient needs to say or to understand.

Patient assessment

When a person presents themselves to a healthcare provider, it is expected that the registered nurse will do the initial assessment. The role of the nursing associate is to provide and monitor the care that has been planned by the nurse (West, 2019). In order to monitor the patient, a continual assessment of the patient needs to be maintained, and this is within the scope of practice of the nursing associate.

Continual nursing assessment is done in a holistic manner, and it is important here to ask the right questions and be able to empathise with the individual patient in front of you to make sure that their needs are responded to. As a nursing associate you will spend time with the patient, enabling you to understand them and make sure that they are treated fairly. You will be able to talk to the patient about any spiritual needs that they may have and get them the support that they may need. You can talk with them about what they need help with and make notes to ensure everyone involved with the patient understands their physical and mental health needs.

In 1980 Roper et al. developed the 'activities of living' (ALs) concept, which serves as a template when performing a holistic assessment of a patient (Roper et al., 2000). This was to enable nurses to step away from the medical model of only looking at a patient's physical symptoms and to consider their whole self in relation to their healthcare. You will see assessment proformas based on the ALs where you work. They include asking the patient certain questions about their everyday life (see Table 7.1).

Table 7.1 Activities of living

Maintaining a safe environment – this can be related to a person's place of residence or related to lifestyle choices.	Personal cleansing and dressing – selecting clothing, being able to wash self and dress self.	Eliminating – bowels and bladder. Ability to self-manage. Assess if any equipment is required.
Communicating – language requirements. Pain levels. Freedom to communicate. To whom they are willing to communicate.	Controlling body temperature – exposure needs to be considered, plus cost of living and impacting illnesses.	Expressing sexuality – what makes the patient feel like themselves – cleanliness, impact of illness and medications.
Breathing – rate, depth, ease. Assess if any equipment is needed.	Mobilising – how independent and for how far.	Sleeping – normal sleeping pattern and any changes.
Eating and drinking – preferences, ability and how food is prepared and by whom.	Working and playing – friends, hobbies, job.	Dying – fears, worries, needs.

The 12 ALs listed in Table 7.1 consider common needs and requirements for all people with any medical condition. However, due to everyone being different, each of the ALs needs to be considered with regard to a person's independence and dependence across the lifespan. The following five factors also need to be considered:

- biological
- psychological
- sociocultural
- environmental
- politico-economical

By assessing each AL alongside each of the five factors, equitable person-centred care can be delivered. It is easy for healthcare professionals to assume that everybody wants to be 'normal', that is, to be independent in all respects, however, that is not everybody's normal and that is important to remember. If you have a patient who runs five times a week and presents with a broken leg, their recovery is going to be psychologically challenging as they may struggle with immobility. A more sedate person who can work from home and whose hobby is playing computer games, for example, is likely to find the recovery from a broken leg less psychologically challenging. There is no such thing as 'normal' when considering a person's quality of life; it is a subjective notion and should never be judged on your own expectations.

Case study: Jo

Jo is 19 years old and has a moderate learning difficulty that enables them to communicate independently, but means they cannot make decisions about their healthcare due to not having the capacity to do so. They have been admitted to hospital as they require an appendicectomy. They are distressed at their level of pain and cannot mobilise well. They are frightened as they have never had an operation before. Jo's parents brought them in. Jo lives with their parents, and they make most decisions for Jo. Jo attends a social day centre which specialises in supporting people with learning difficulties and Jo has many friends there. Jo's favourite subjects are science and art. Jo also enjoys gardening.

Activity 7.2   Reflection

- What needs to be taken into consideration when assessing Jo?
- What would help to ensure Jo's rights are always protected while they are in hospital?
- Are there special adjustments that will need to be made for Jo's stay in hospital?
- Thinking about the ALs, what main issues seem to arise from this case study?

An outline answer is provided at the end of the chapter.

Case study: Adam

Adam is a 56-year-old man who was diagnosed with young-onset dementia eight years ago. Adam has been admitted due to sustaining a fall and fracturing his left hip. An ambulance was called for him by a passer-by. Adam lives in a two-storey three-bedroom house with his wife. His only child is at a university four hours away. His wife works full time. She is Adam's health and welfare attorney. Adam no longer drives but does go out for short walks every day. At times Adam is slightly confused but this seems to be when he is in an unfamiliar environment. He is safe at home by himself during the day and in his local area as he knows where he is. He is independent with his day-to-day needs at home. On admission to the ward in which you work the nurse notes that Adam is disorientated and frightened and this is making him verbally aggressive towards the nursing team. He is asking for his wife, but he does not know her phone number and his distress is making it difficult for him to be able to answer the questions that he is asked during his assessment. He does have a card in his wallet, which gives his personal details. When asked to consent to surgery he refuses as he states that he doesn't want to die in hospital and that he wants to go home and that his wife will look after him there.

Activity 7.3   Reflection

- What needs to be taken into consideration when assessing Adam?
- What would help to ensure Adam's rights are always protected while he is in hospital?
- Are there special adjustments that will need to be made for Adam's stay in hospital?
- Thinking about the ALs, what main issues seem to arise from this case study?

An outline answer is provided at the end of the chapter.

Figure 7.1 depicts Roper, Logan and Tierney's model of nursing, showing how all of the elements work together when assessing a patient.

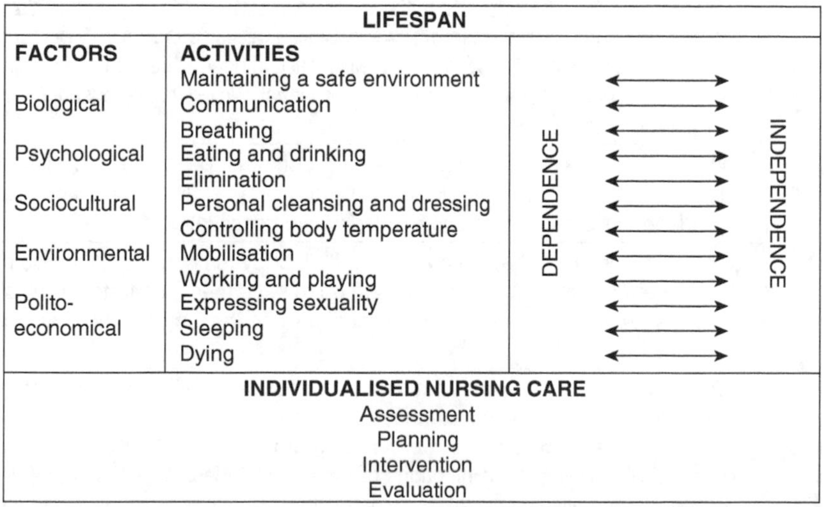

Figure 7.1   Roper, Logan and Tierney's model of nursing (adapted from Roper et al., 2000)

ALs occur every day for every person, which is why, when performing the continued assessment of a patient, it is important to understand the diverse needs of the patient for each of the ALs. Some of the factors are outlined in Table 7.2.

Table 7.2 ALs and EDI considerations

Activity	Things to consider with regard to EDI
Maintaining a safe environment	People have different ideas of what is and what is not maintaining a safe environment. People make choices that could be judged as being unwise, like drinking alcohol, eating certain foods, taking drugs or doing certain sports. However, everyone has the right to live the way that they want to. Healthcare professionals cannot judge what may have been the cause of the ill health for that patient.
	Some people cannot live in a safe environment. They may not have enough money to look after themselves properly. They may be homeless or live in overcrowded housing due to their economic status. They may be in an abusive relationship or be being exploited. Healthcare professionals don't always hear the backstory of the patient, so judgements about them must not be made.
Communicating	Different cultures have different ways of communicating. As well as language barriers there may be some situations where, for a variety of reasons, a female cannot speak directly to a male.
	There are also communication differences, such as when someone has a hearing or sight impairment. Children also communicate differently to adults.
	Some people may speak the same language as you but in a different way which makes it hard to understand or work with.
	It is the responsibility of the healthcare provider to understand their patients and to explain things to them in a way that they can understand (Mental Capacity Act 2005).
Breathing	Some people have asthma or other conditions which impact breathing. Some people smoke and that impacts their breathing. Some people are overweight, which can impact their breathing.
Eating and drinking	Eating and drinking are fundamental to society. They present an opportunity for people to socialise, celebrate and comfort themselves. Through food and drink people also show their love for someone else. When someone is unwell, families often want to feed them to provide comfort. Sometimes this is ill-advised from a medical perspective and this needs to be explained to everyone as that can be upsetting.
Eliminating	Some people do not discuss their bowel habits as this is seen as a very personal subject. Unfortunately, it is something we prioritise in healthcare, so making someone feel comfortable when talking about this is essential. We do that by ensuring privacy and maintaining dignity.
Personal cleansing and dressing	When someone is ill they can become reliant on other people to help with personal cleansing and dressing. The 'sick role' (Morton et al., 2020) is important to understand, as independence should be encouraged where possible.
Controlling body temperature	When someone is ill, they cannot control their body temperature. When someone is ill, family members may want to wrap them up to keep them comfortable, which may not be advisable in that situation. Communication with the family is important to promote the best patient care.
Mobilisation	When someone is ill they may not prioritise mobilisation. For some patients, getting out of their bed is too much and they don't want to walk around the ward. However, they should be encouraged to in order to promote independence and prevent other conditions like chest infections or pressure injuries. When someone does not want to mobilise themselves, it is important to explain its importance and offer encouragement. They cannot be forced to due to their autonomy.

Activity	Things to consider with regard to EDI
Working and playing	Everyone has different priorities. Some people have children, some people have pets, some people have jobs that they feel they cannot leave. Some people are only paid when they work. Being ill can impact on all of these things and this can affect the recovery of the patient. The patient may not be able to accept the care that they need if they have other priorities that they feel unable to change.
Expressing sexuality	There are many challenges for patients when expressing their sexuality. Some patients may find it challenging to inform their carers if they are LGBTQIA+ for example. Some healthcare professionals do not act professionally around certain patients, for example, consistently referring to a transgender person with the wrong pronoun or the wrong name.
Sleeping	People need different amounts of sleep. There are different thoughts on how much sleep is 'ideal' but different people manage on different amounts. Too much or too little can be detrimental to that individual's health. When in hospital it is not expected that people will sleep well, which is known to be detrimental to healing and this does need to be taken into consideration.
Dying	End-of-life care is very personal and complex, and it is explored later in this chapter.

When a healthcare professional asks a patient personal questions it is expected that the patient will tell the truth, but sometimes they do not for a variety of reasons. This is why effective communication skills are so important and they may help the patient to trust you and tell you all that you need to know.

As a nursing associate you do not complete the initial assessment of a patient, however, you are expected to provide continuing care and continual assessments, so it is important that you understand the complexity of a holistic assessment.

One activity of living that doesn't happen every day is dying. However, it is important that person-centred care is prioritised when someone is dying. This section explains some specific end-of-life customs for certain cultures that you should be aware of.

Religious beliefs in end-of-life care

When someone is at the end of their life, their preferences, their beliefs and their personal needs are more important than ever. Working with dying people is a privilege for healthcare workers, and it is important to get things right. Sudden, unexpected deaths can be traumatic for everyone involved, but an expected death for someone can be managed in a way that is not traumatic. This requires careful planning with the patient and their family to ensure that person-centred needs are met as much as possible.

This section will look at a selection of different cultural requirements at the end of life.

According to the 2021 Census, 46.2 per cent of people in England and Wales describe themselves as Christian, 6.5 per cent are Muslim, 1.7 per cent are Hindu, 0.5 per cent are Jewish, 0.9 per cent are Sikh, 0.6 per cent have other religions, while 37.2 per cent describe themselves as having no religion. You will look after patients from different backgrounds during your career and it is important that you know how to find out what their specific needs are.

Christianity

Christianity generally is holding a belief in Jesus Christ, but within Christianity there are many different specific faiths, including Anglicans, Roman Catholic, Eastern Orthodoxy, Protestantism, Presbyterian, Methodists, Baptists, Quakers, Jehovah's Witnesses and Mormons plus many more. The needs at the end of life will vary depending on the specific religion of the practising

Christian. For example, Catholics may ask to have the Sacrament of the Sick (or Last Rights as they are often known) whereas Protestants may want prayers and communion at their bedside. Baptising infants at risk of dying may be important for both Catholics and Protestants. As a nursing associate you need to be aware of different requirements for Christians.

Hinduism

Hindu belief teaches that the state of mind at death is important so there should be an atmosphere that reminds the person of their relationship with God, such as pictures of saints, special sacred flowers and rosary beads. An issue that may affect you as a nursing associate is that it is traditional that family members come to visit the dying person to show respect, to ask forgiveness for any offences that may have occurred, and to say goodbye. This may mean a lot of people visiting, which needs to be managed by the nursing team. A practical solution for this may be working with the immediate family to negotiate a limit to how many people visit at any one time.

Islam

Islamic practice is to pray five times a day, facing Mecca. A dying Muslim may ask to face Mecca in order to pray, which may not be possible depending on the room that they are in, so their bed allocation needs to be considered. Muslims can only pray when they are clean, so healthcare workers need to be aware of that requirement and support the patient as much as possible. Muslims often make decisions as a whole family and confidentiality needs to be respected by asking the patient who they would like information shared with. People who follow Islam need to be buried within 24 hours of death, which is not always possible depending upon the circumstances of the death. If a postmortem is needed, then the burial can be delayed.

Buddhism

Buddhists believe in mindfulness, so dying with a clear mind may be of importance to them. This may impact their willingness to take certain medication. Buddhism teaches that, once a heart stops beating, it can take some time until that person is fully dead. The deceased person should not be touched or moved to allow them to complete their journey for at least four hours following their death. It is important to not touch the patient's head and only wash the body where it is essential. An understanding of this will help your role as a nursing associate when caring for a Buddhist at the end of their life.

Judaism

Jewish people cannot pray if they are not clean, but it is not always acceptable for the healthcare worker to wash the patient. It is important to ask the relatives how much intervention they would like. A dying person of the Jewish faith should not be left alone, and neither should the dead body. But as it is impractical for a healthcare worker to stay with a dying person continually, a family member can stay with them. Once the person has died, it is not possible for a family member to stay with the dead body in the hospital and this needs to be explained.

Sikhism

As death becomes close, a person of Sikh faith may want to be surrounded by friends and family. Sikh scriptures need to be recited constantly to allow the dying person to focus on their God and not on worldly matters in order for their souls to be reborn. This requirement could impact their care delivery, so you need to have an understanding of it in order to work with the family to ensure the best care is given to the patient at all times, while respecting their right to religion.

Of course, these are just guidelines because every person will have their own specific needs, for example, although a patient might identify as Catholic, they may not be a practising Catholic and therefore not want the last rights. However, their family might feel very strongly about it, so they may choose to have the blessing to help soothe their family. Some people do not have a religion but are spiritual and have specific requirements at the end of life.

You are not expected to know all the needs and requirements of all of the different patients you may come across, but you are expected to know that there are differences and that you should ask someone what they would like by using your communication skills. That ensures you are delivering person-centred, culturally competent care. Some further reading to help you improve your knowledge is included at the end of this chapter.

Activity 7.4   Reflection

- What spiritual services are available in your place of work?
- Do you have access to a chaplain or a priest?
- Many hospitals have someone who comes in every day – do you have that? If so, what denomination are they?
- How easy is it to get someone from a non-traditional Christian faith?

As this activity is based on your own observation, no outline answer is provided at the end of the chapter.

Chapter summary

This chapter has considered the importance of respecting each patient that you meet and remembering that each person has individual needs and values. It is important to give people time to make decisions and to respect the decisions that they make. Assessment was explored with consideration given to some of the individual factors that need to be taken into account for each patient.

Activities: Brief outline answers

Activity 7.2

1. Jo is over the age of 18 but is unable to consent for themselves. However, they don't have a power of attorney, so the medical team has to work in the best interests of Jo, with the support of the parents. Asking the parents what they believe Jo would want is important in this situation as it maintains person-centred care and ensures Jo's best interests are paramount.

2. Keeping constant communication both with Jo and Jo's parents is essential. Jo must be allowed to be heard and to express opinions with Jo's parents overseeing. Jo's rights must be respected at all times.

3. Jo should be on an adult ward but it may be more appropriate for them to be on a children's ward depending on the policy of that hospital. If they stay on an adult ward then a parent may also need to stay, which would be unusual in an adult ward.

4. The ALs need to be assessed holistically, taking into consideration the current needs of Jo and Jo's age. This is outlined in the following table.

Maintaining a safe environment – Jo may not be able to maintain a safe environment independently. This may be a long-term issue or an acute one.	Personal cleansing and dressing – Jo should be able to do some self-care but may need support, especially while in pain.	Eliminating – Jo may usually be independent with elimination needs, but due to the high pain levels may need support.
Communicating – Jo may struggle to express themselves due to the high pain level and fear of being in hospital. Jo's parents may be the only people who can really understand Jo, so they need to be available to provide reassurance and clarity.	Controlling body temperature – Jo is unable to control this due to the appendicitis.	Expressing sexuality – It is unclear how Jo is feeling about themselves right now but they won't be feeling comfortable due to the appendicitis.
Breathing – Fear and pain will impact Jo's breathing rate and depth.	Mobilising – Jo is unable to mobilise due to the pain, which is unusual for them.	Sleeping – Jo will not be able to sleep due to the pain, which will impact their wellbeing.
Eating and drinking – Jo will be nil by mouth prior to surgery so may be hungry and may not fully understand why they cannot eat or drink. Jo may have particular food needs and this would need to be discussed with their parents.	Working and playing – Jo is going through a different experience due to needing surgery and this means they cannot do what they would normally enjoy doing. This will have an impact on their health as they will also need recovery time.	Dying – Jo may be fearful of death due to needing surgery and everything will need to be explained very clearly in order to manage the fear and worry.

There may be other issues that you picked up from the case scenario and your own practice experiences to add to those documented here.

Activity 7.3

1. When assessing Adam it is important to perform a mental capacity assessment to decide if he can make decisions for himself or not. People with dementia often have times of complete clarity, so it is important to not assume anything about Adam when caring for him.

2. If Adam is assessed as having capacity then his decision to not have surgery should be heard and all options explained to him fully. If he does not have capacity then his wife needs to be called as his power of attorney to make that decision in his best interests.

3. Adam has young-onset dementia and becomes disoriented when he is somewhere unfamiliar, so items from home could be brought in to make his bed area feel more familiar to him. A communication passport would be helpful for the staff looking after Adam to understand how to help to prevent him becoming upset.

4. Adam, despite his diagnosis, remains independent but this surgery will change his position on the continuum and this will impact his day-to-day life. The ALs outlined in the following table need to be considered with the intention of returning Adam to his independent levels as soon as possible:

Maintaining a safe environment – Adam is in a new environment and he is disorientated. This increases his risks of trips and falls.	Personal cleansing and dressing – Adam is usually independent with his personal hygiene needs, but post surgery he will need assistance. His wife works full time so discharge planning needs to consider who will help Adam.	Eliminating – Adam is usually independent with his elimination needs but the analgesia he will be on may impact his bowel movements and he may not be able to use the toilet independently post surgery.
Communicating – Adam is not able to communicate effectively due to being disorientated.	Controlling body temperature – Adam is in hospital, which may be at a different temperature to his home environment. He does not have an infection but is responding to the fractured hip so may not be able to control his temperature.	Expressing sexuality – Adam is asking for his wife. Due to the disorientation he may not feel like himself or have confidence in his own cognitive ability at this time.
Breathing – Adam is likely to be in pain which will impact his breathing.	Mobilising – Adam will not be able to mobilise independently post surgery, which will impact his ability to be on his own at home while his wife is at work.	Sleeping – Adam may struggle to sleep due to pain levels both pre and post surgery.
Eating and drinking – Adam usually manages his own food during the day but this will be difficult for him post surgery.	Working and playing – Adam doesn't work but does go out every day and this will be challenging post surgery. This is going to impact his wellbeing.	Dying – As he is in a hospital, Adam may be scared that he is going to die. He should be reassured about the care that he is being given.

There may be other issues that you picked up from the case scenario and your own practice experiences to add to those documented here.

Further reading

Public Health England (2016) *Faith at End of Life.* Available at: **www.gov.uk/government/publications/faith-at-end-of-life-public-health-approach-resource-for-professionals**

This document offers guidance on different religious requirements at the end of life.

Pentaris, P and Tripathi, K (2022) Palliative professionals' views on the importance of religion, belief, and spiritual identities toward the end of life. *International Journal of Environmental Research and Public Health,* 19(10): 6031. Available at: **www.ncbi.nlm.nih.gov/pmc/articles/PMC9141656/**

This article gives different perspectives on the personal priorities for end-of-life care.

Camara, C and Rosengarten, L (2021) Faith-sensitive end of life care for children, young people and their families. *British Journal of Nursing.* Available at: **www.britishjournalofnursing.com/content/clinical/faith-sensitive-end-of-life-care-for-children-young-people-and-their-families/**

This article focuses on specific religions and highlights the importance of understanding faith in end-of-life care.

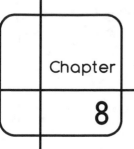

Application of EDI to practice

Chapter aims

After reading this chapter, you will be able to:

- explore different clinical examples to apply the theory of EDI to practice;
- discuss when reasonable adjustments are appropriate and when they are not;
- apply legal and ethical decision-making to clinical situations;
- maintain person-centred care in complex clinical situations.

Introduction

As seen throughout this book, applying EDI is an important element of person-centred care. This chapter will consider various scenarios and case studies to explore the principles of respecting EDI in healthcare in more depth. It will use specific examples where differences need to be understood in order for adjustments to be made. It will also consider situations where respecting a person's culture and beliefs is not possible and explore why. The Equality Act and the Human Rights Act will be applied to complex clinical situations, as will some ethical considerations to help guide how best to provide person-centred care.

Case study: The Paul family

A family of four are in a road traffic accident and are taken to A & E. There is Richard Paul, a 41-year-old male, Christina Paul, a 15-year-old female, and Thomas Paul, a 6-year-old male. They are all bleeding and are likely to need blood transfusions to survive. The mother, Fran Paul, a 39-year-old female, was in the accident but is not as badly injured as the rest of her family. She explains that they are all Jehovah's Witnesses and none of them want a blood transfusion.

As is well known, people who are of the Jehovah's Witness faith do not believe in having blood transfusions as their Bible, the New World Translation of the Holy Scriptures, states that people must not 'eat' blood as the blood represents life. This is interpreted as not being able to accept blood transfusions. Unfortunately, this can have an impact on their recovery and could even lead to their death, but this is something that a Jehovah's Witness knows and understands.

This is a challenging situation for the healthcare team.

Things to consider

Firstly, it is essential to respect the family's right to autonomy and their protected right to religion. This is protected by the Human Rights Act and the Equality Act. No one is in a position to judge them and their choices. People have a right to refuse any treatment for any reason at all and as healthcare professionals the responsibility is to advocate for the patient and protect their rights. The 41-year-old male has a right to refuse any blood products as he is over 18 and can make that decision. Remember, decisions do not have to be considered 'wise' to be valid. The 15-year-old is slightly different as she is under the age of 18, but, if it can be shown that she is Gillick competent (see 'Understanding the theory' box), then her right to refuse must be respected. The case of the 6-year-old is different again. The child's parents have the responsibility of making his decisions at this time and they want to refuse to let him have a transfusion on religious grounds. However, the right to life is also a human right and no one should be deprived of their life intentionally. In this situation the medical team may give him a transfusion in order to save his life without the consent of his parents by working in his best interests, as allowing him to die when he could be saved is not. This is permitted in law under the Children Act of 1989 as explored in Chapter 4.

The protection of life is a legal requirement and a priority for healthcare workers, but if there is a way to protect life that doesn't defy a person's religion, then that way should be explored.

Understanding the theory: Gillick competency

In Chapter 2 autonomy and capacity were explored and it was explained that a person under the age of 16 will not be able to consent for themselves. However, under the Gillick competency decision of 1984, they may be able to. If a young person is found to understand the treatment offered to them, including the side effects, the risks and the likely result, then they can consent to or refuse the treatment offered. The ability to do this may depend on the treatment offered and some situations may be too complex, and, as with capacity in adults, the ability to consent can fluctuate. If a Gillick-competent child accepts treatment the medical team will support this decision. If a child chooses to refuse treatment this decision can be overridden by a medical team on the basis that the young person may not fully understand the treatment offered (CQC, 2022). You may feel that this is unfair as, unlike adult consent, a Gillick-competent child may be found unable to make a decision about their treatment because the decision is considered unwise, and therefore they may not fully understand the situation. An adult is not judged in the same way and it is clear that a decision does not need to be wise to have been made with capacity. But with a child, if they are making a decision that is against medical advice then it can be assumed that they do not have capacity because of their age.

Case study: Visiting policy

You are working in a hospice and a patient under your care is at the end stage of their life. The family has been informed that this person has just 24 to 48 hours left to live. You are asked if family members can come to sit with them. You say yes and explain that the hospice does not have specific visitor restrictions like hospitals do. The family is clearly relieved and grateful that you will allow other members of the family to visit. Two hours later, 37 people come into the hospice and you are informed that as part of the travelling community culture all family members are expected to be with their loved one when they die.

Due to the large number of people, the situation becomes loud and disruptive for the rest of the patients in that bay and other patients and families in the hospice become upset and complain. The other patients would like a more restful environment while they are at the end of their lives and having this number of people there is preventing that. This is distressing for all involved.

Things to consider

The travelling community need their rituals to be respected. Their rights are protected under the Human Rights Act and the Equality Act. But the other patients and relatives feel that allowing 37 people to stand vigil is invasive and overwhelming, and is causing them distress at a stressful time when their rights need to be respected. Looking at the justice element of this situation it is difficult to maintain fairness for all of the parties involved. The culture of the travelling community should be respected, but not at the expense of the other patients. Equity is about fairness for all, not just for one patient and their family. A way to manage all of the needs of all of the patients is essential, and moving your patient into a side room to give the family easier access and more privacy or giving the family a space elsewhere to be together and asking them to take turns to sit with the patient, might present the best-case scenarios in this situation.

Case study: Force-feeding babies

There are practices that are acceptable in some countries but not in the country in which you are working. For example, in countries like Ghana (and others), it is sometimes the practice to pour food into the mouth of a baby using a funnel to ensure that the baby swallows all of the food. It is believed that this process will help the baby put on weight and therefore thrive (Wrottesley et al., 2020). However, force-feeding a child is dangerous as the food can aspirate into the child's lungs and cause severe health issues.

According to the BBC (2023), in 2011 Gloria Dwoma, a nurse originally from Ghana, was convicted of causing or allowing the death of her baby due to force-feeding it using a funnel and causing it to develop pneumonia through the aspiration of food. She claimed she was simply following the practice of her own mother and family and was only trying to make sure her baby was fed well. She was given a three-year custodial sentence.

Her right to a personal and family life is absolute (Human Rights Act 1998), but causing the death of her baby is against the law in England. While she has a right to her cultural practices, they are not acceptable under English law. She did not mean to harm her child but as a registered nurse working in the UK it was felt that she should have also known the harm that she was causing and she was therefore found guilty. She was responsible for keeping her baby safe but, instead, her actions caused the baby's death.

Case study: Patients who want to request specific people to care for them

When admitted to an inpatient setting, many patients need to have members of the healthcare team perform personal care on them. This can be embarrassing for the patient, or it can be intimidating for them. It can make a patient feel uncomfortable and vulnerable. A patient may make a request that only certain members of the team look after them, and this could be due to the perceived gender, race or sexuality of that person. For example, a patient may only want Caucasian healthcare workers to look after them, or they might only want heterosexual healthcare workers or only female healthcare workers to administer their care.

Things to consider

Legally there is nothing that states that patients can demand which nurses and nursing associates look after them and which ones do not, and such requests would contravene the Equality Act and the NHS zero tolerance of abuse to staff policy. However, in order to promote patient-centred care, it is considered good practice to make reasonable adjustments to meet any requests made, and the Human Rights Act does give everyone the right to decide what happens to their body. For example, as a healthcare worker you do not know if a patient has a history of being abused, and this is perhaps why they want only female staff looking after them. Or there could be another reason such as a religious requirement. Similarly, requesting a nurse who speaks the same language as the patient is not unreasonable, although it may not be possible to provide.

However, the patient with racial preferences presents a different problem here, as the NHS has a zero-tolerance policy on racial abuse of its staff, so abiding with the patient request could be considered to contravene that policy. Similarly, homophobic patients also present challenges, as meeting their needs would go against the policy of the acceptance of LGBTQIA+ within the NHS. Sometimes to protect the staff member from abuse it may be wise to not put healthcare workers from an ethnic minority with a potentially racist patient or LGBTQIA+ healthcare workers with a potentially homophobic patient. Although it may feel like the prejudice is being rewarded, if that action protects the staff from abuse, then it may be a necessary step to take.

By listening to the patient's requests and reacting to their needs, the relationship with that patient will be preserved and trust may be promoted, which will have a positive impact on that patient. It may also make them more concordant with the care being offered and delivered as they are more comfortable.

Activity 8.1 Reflection

There are some religions that require that each gender only be touched by people of the same gender (unless they are close family). Therefore, their religion requires that they are nursed by people of the same gender as themselves. This requirement should be protected as it is a religious one, but from a practical perspective this can be really challenging. However, considering that only 11 per cent of registered nurses identify as male (NMC, 2023c), this requirement might be difficult to fulfil, but it is the patient's right to request it and it should be abided by as much as is practicable. Consider the following:

- What is the male to female ratio where you work?
- Would it be possible for a male patient to always have a male nurse or nursing associate providing all their care at any time of day on any day of the week?

As this activity is a personal reflection, no outline answer is provided at the end of the chapter.

When reasonable adjustments are not reasonable

There are practices that are acceptable and normal in some countries but are not acceptable in England, and as a nursing associate you are obliged to report certain things as non-acceptable practice. The list shown in Table 8.1 is non-exhaustive but provides a few examples.

Table 8.1 Controversial practices

Female genital mutilation (FGM)	FGM is the process of either partially or completely removing female genitalia for no medical reason. It is carried out on females aged between 0 and 15 and practised in 30 countries in Africa, the Middle East and Asia. It is recognised internationally as a violation of human rights against women and if identified or suspected, must be reported to the police (WHO, 2023).
Conversion therapy	Conversion therapy is a 'treatment' for LGBTQIA+ people to try to make them heterosexual. Many countries have banned this therapy (in adolescents if not adults) but as of November 2023 England has not. Ministers have proposed it be banned, but this has yet to come into effect. While you cannot report conversion therapy to the police, being the patient's advocate is your role and you need to offer the patient all options that are available to them.
Euthanasia/ assisted suicide	New Zealand, Australia, Canada, Switzerland, The Netherlands, Belgium, Luxembourg and, in the USA, Oregon, Washington and California have all legalised either euthanasia or assisted dying for people who are suffering. The United Kingdom has not legalised euthanasia or assisted dying. Euthanasia is considered murder in England and if someone is found guilty of helping someone to die from suicide, they may be imprisoned for up to 14 years. There are various organisations asking for a change in the law, but, as it stands, the government has not yet put forward a bill.

Empathy

The most important thing to remember when looking after anyone is to be kind, to try to understand their perspective and to respect their needs. The ability to put someone else's needs before your own without judgement is essential in healthcare and this is part of being an empathetic practitioner. To be person-centred and to act as the patient's advocate, you need to be empathetic to all of your patients. You may not always understand their needs and wants but your job is not to judge. Your job is to listen and imagine what they are going through. Remember, no two people will have the exact same experience as each other and you will never really understand what someone is feeling. But you can empathise with them. You can imagine you are them and consider their needs and thoughts instead of your own. If you do this then you will provide fair, unbiased, patient-centred care.

The role of the nursing associate

The cases explored in this chapter are complex and would require input from many members of the multidisciplinary team. As a nursing associate you may struggle to see what your role is in these situations. You must always work within your scope of practice, but your Standards of Proficiency do state that you must advocate for patients to ensure non-discriminatory, person-centred care. The Standards also tell you to work as part of the multidisciplinary team.

Chapter summary

As a nursing associate it is important that you have a good understanding of the personal requirements of the patients in your care. You will not know everything about everyone, but you are well placed to learn about them through talking with your patients and their representatives to develop your understanding. By listening and learning you will be culturally competent and able to deliver person-centred care to all of your patients.

Useful websites

www.dignityindying.org.uk

Dignity in Dying is an organisation that is advocating an assisted dying bill.

www.stonewall.org.uk

Stonewall is an organisation campaigning for the rights of LGBTQIA+ people.

Bibliography

Adigun, O, Mikhail, A, Krawiec, C and Hatcher, J (2023) *Abuse and Neglect*. St Petersburg, FL: StatPearls.

Afriyie, D (2020) Effective communication between nurses and patients: an evolutionary concept analysis. *The British Journal of Community Nursing*, 25(9): 438–45.

Alabi, J (2015) Racial microaggressions in academic libraries: results of a survey of minority and non-minority librarians. *Journal of Academic Librarianship*, 41(1): 47–53.

Alexander, L and Moore, M (2021) 'Deontological ethics', in Edward N. Zalta (ed) *The Stanford Encyclopedia of Philosophy* (Winter 2021 edn). Available at: https://plato.stanford.edu/archives/win2021/entries/ethics-deontological/

Anca, C and Aragon, S (2018) The 3 types of diversity that shape our identities. *Harvard Business Review*, May 24.

Baines, E (2022) Nurse whistleblower who was wrongfully dismissed wins £460k payout. *Nursing Times*. Available at: www.nursingtimes.net/news/community-news/nurse-whistleblower-who-was-wrongfully-dismissed-wins-460k-pay-out-17-06-2022/ (accessed 7 November 2023).

BBC News (2023) Baby force-feeding death: mother Gloria Dwomoh jailed. Available at: www.bbc.co.uk/news/uk-england-london-15689864 (accessed 19 August 2023).

Beauchamp, T and Childress, J (2019) *Principles of Biomedical Ethics* (8th edn). Oxford: Oxford University Press.

Bennett, M (1986) Developmental model of intercultural sensitivity. Available at: https://organizingengagement.org/models/developmental-model-of-intercultural-sensitivity/ (accessed 1 November 2023).

Bolam v *Friern Hospital Management Committee* (1957) 1 WLR 583.

Bolitho v *Hackney HA* (1997) UKHL 46.

Brueck, M and Sulmasy, D (2020) The rule of double effect: a tool for moral deliberation in practice and policy. Harvard, MA: Centre for Bioethics, Harvard Medical School.

Care Quality Commission (CQC) (2011) Mental Capacity Act 2005: guidance for providers. Available at: www.cqc.org.uk/sites/default/files/documents/rp_poc1b2b_100563_20111223_v4_00_guidance_for_providers_mca_for_external_publication.pdf (accessed 7 November 2023).

Care Quality Commission (CQC) (2017) Regulation 20: duty of candour. London: Care Quality Commission. Available at: www.cqc.org.uk/guidance-providers/regulations-enforcement/regulation-20-duty-candour (accessed 7 November 2023).

Care Quality Commission (2022) GP mythbuster 8: Gillick competency and Fraser guidelines. Available at: www.cqc.org.uk/guidance-providers/gps/gp-mythbusters/gp-mythbuster-8-gillick-competency-fraser-guidelines (accessed 1 November 2023).

Chester v *Afshar* (2004) UKHL 41.

Children Act 1989, c. 31. Available at: www.legislation.gov.uk/ukpga/2004/31/contents (accessed 26 July 2023).

Choudry, M, Latif, A and Warburton, K (2018) An overview of the spiritual importance of end-of-life care among the five major faiths of the United Kingdom. *Clinical Medicine,* 18(1): 23–31.

Coulter, A and Collins, A (2011) Making shared decision-making a reality: no decision about me without me. London: The Kings Fund.

Coulter, A and Oldham, J (2016) Person-centred care: what is it and how do we get there? *Future Hospital Journal,* 3(2): 114–16.

Council of Europe (1950) European Convention for the Protection of Human Rights and Fundamental Freedoms, as amended by Protocols Nos. 11 and 14, 4 November 1950, ETS 5. Available at: www.refworld.org/docid/3ae6b3b04.html (accessed 24 February 2023).

DHSC (Department of Health and Social Care) Media Centre (2023) NHS workforce: record numbers of doctors and nurses in NHS. Available at: https://healthmedia.blog.gov.uk/2023/04/27/nhs-workforce-record-numbers-of-doctors-and-nurses-in-nhs/ (accessed 27 April 2023).

Einstein, A (1952) in Kelly, M (2004) *The Rhythm of Life: Living Every Day with Passion and Purpose.* New York: Fireside.

Equality Act 2010. Available at: Available at: www.opsi.gov.uk/acts/acts2010/ukpga-20100015-en-1 (accessed 24 February 2023).

Firdous, T, Darwin, Z and Hassan, SM (2020) Muslim women's experiences of maternity services in the UK: qualitative systematic review and thematic synthesis. *BMC Pregnancy and Childbirth,* 20(115).

Francis, R (2013) *Report of the Mid Staffordshire NHS Foundation Trust Public Inquiry.* London: Robert Francis.

Gillon, R (2003) Ethics needs principles – four can encompass the rest – and respect for autonomy should be 'first among equals'. *Journal of Medical Ethics,* 29(5): 307–12.

Gonzalez, D, Bethencourt Mirabal, A and McCall, JD (2023) Child abuse and neglect. [Updated 2023 July 4], in StatPearls [Internet]. Treasure Island, FL: StatPearls Publishing; 2023, Jan–. Available at: www.ncbi.nlm.nih.gov/books/NBK459146/ (accessed 23 May 2023).

Gopal, D, Chetty, U, O'Donnell, P, Gajria, C and Blackadder-Weinstein, J (2021) Implicit bias in healthcare: clinical practice, research and decision-making. *Future Healthcare Journal,* 8(1): 40–8.

GOV.UK (2007) The Department for Constitutional Affairs (2007) The Mental Capacity Act 2005 Code of Practice. United Kingdom: Crown Copyright.

GOV.UK (2010) No health without mental health. Available at: https://assets.publishing.service.gov.uk/media/5a7c348ae5274a25a914129d/dh_124058.pdf (accessed 29 December 2022).

GOV.UK (2015, updated 2022) All our health: personalised care and population health. Available at: www.gov.uk/government/collections/all-our-health-personalised-care-and-population-health (accessed 29 December 2022).

GOV.UK (2019) New national strategy to tackle Gypsy, Roma and Traveller inequalities. Available at: www.gov.uk/government/news/new-national-strategy-to-tackle-gypsy-roma-and-traveller-inequalities (accessed 29 December 2022).

GOV.UK (2020a) Employing prisoners and ex-offenders. Available at: www.gov.uk/government/publications/unlock-opportunity-employer-information-pack-and-case-studies/employing-prisoners-and-ex-offenders (accessed 29 December 2022).

GOV.UK (2020b) NHS workforce. Available at: www.ethnicity-facts-figures.service.gov.uk/workforce-and-business/workforce-diversity/nhs-workforce/latest (accessed 29 October 2022).

GOV.UK (2021a) Independent report health. Available at: www.gov.uk/government/publications/the-report-of-the-commission-on-race-and-ethnic-disparities/health (accessed 24 July 2023).

GOV.UK (2021b) Writing about ethnicity. Available at: www.ethnicity-facts-figures.service.gov.uk/style-guide/writing-about-ethnicity (accessed 24 July 2023).

GOV.UK (2022) Inclusion health: applying all our health. Available at: www.gov.uk/government/publications/inclusion-health-applying-all-our-health/inclusion-health-applying-all-our-health (accessed 29 December 2022).

GOV.UK (2023a) The NHS Constitution for England. Available at: www.gov.uk/government/publications/the-nhs-constitution-for-england (accessed 24 February 2023).

GOV.UK (2023b) Legislative process: taking a bill through Parliament. Available at: www.gov.uk/guidance/legislative-process-taking-a-bill-through-parliament (accessed 7 November 2023).

Government Equalities Office (2018) National LGBT Survey: summary report. Available at: https://assets.publishing.service.gov.uk/media/5b3cb6b6ed915d39fd5f14df/GEO-LGBT-Survey-Report.pdf (accessed 29 December 2022).

Greenfields, M and Brindley, M (2016) Impact of insecure accommodation and the living environment on Gypsies' and Travellers' health. London: Traveller Movement and Buckinghamshire New University.

Hanif, W and Susarla, R (2018) Diabetes and cardiovascular risk in UK South Asians: an overview. *British Journal of Cardiology*, 25(suppl 2): S8–S13.

Ho, FK, Gray, SR, Welsh, P, Gill, JMR, Sattar, N, Pell, JP and Celis-Morales, C (2022) Ethnic differences in cardiovascular risk: examining differential exposure and susceptibility to risk factors. *BMC Medicine*, 20(1): 149.

Hoffman, KM, Trawaltera, S, Axta, J and Norman Oliver, M (2016) Racial bias in pain assessment and treatment recommendations, and false beliefs about biological differences between blacks and whites. *PNAS*, 113(16): 4296–301.

Hoffman, K, Trawalter, S, Axt, J and Oliver, M (2016) Racial bias in pain assessment and treatment recommendations, and false beliefs about biological differences between blacks and whites. *Proceedings of the National Academy of Science of the United States of America*, 113(16): 4296–301.

House of Commons (2011) How laws are made. Available at: www.parliament.uk/globalassets/documents/commons-information-office/easy-read-guides/easy-read-laws.pdf (accessed 1 November 2023).

Human Rights Act 1998. Available at: www.legislation.gov.uk/ukpga/1998/42/schedule/1 (accessed 23 February 2023).

Kelly, M (2004) *The Rhythm of Life: Living Every Day with Passion and Purpose.* New York: Fireside.

Lee, A (2017) 'Bolam' to 'Montgomery' is a result of evolutionary change of medical practice towards 'patient-centred care'. *Postgraduate Medical Journal,* 93(1095): 46–50.

MacLellan, J, Collins, S, Myatt, M, Pope, C, Knighton, W and Rai, T (2022) Black, Asian and minority ethnic women's experiences of maternity services in the UK: a qualitative evidence synthesis. *Journal of Advanced Nursing,* 78: 2175–90.

Marcelin, J, Siraj, D, Victor, R, Kotadia, S and Maldonado, Y (2019) The impact of unconscious bias in healthcare: how to recognize and mitigate it. *The Journal of Infectious Diseases,* 220: S62–73.

Mental Capacity Act 2005. Available at: www.legislation.gov.uk/ukpga/2005/9/pdfs/ukpga_20050009_en.pdf (accessed 24 February 2023).

Mental Health Act 1983. Available at: www.legislation.gov.uk/ukpga/1983/20/contents (accessed 7 November 2023).

Moffat, P (2021) Has sexism in the NHS become normalised? *Journal of Health Visiting,* 9: 9.

Montgomery v Lanarkshire Health Board (1995) UKSC 1.

Morton, L, Cogan, N, Kornfalt, S, Porter, Z and Georgiadis, E (2020) Baring all: the impact of the hospital gown on patient well-being. *British Journal of Health Psychology,* 25(3): 452–73.

Myers, V (2016) in Cho, J 'Diversity is being invited to the party; inclusion is being asked to dance,' Verna Myers tells Cleveland Bar. Available at: www.cleveland.com/business/2016/05/diversity_is_being_invited_to.html (accessed 1 November 2023).

NHLBI (The National Heart, Lung and Blood Institute) (2017) Opioid crisis adds to pain of sickle cell patients. Available at: www.nhlbi.nih.gov/news/2017/opioid-crisis-adds-pain-sickle-cell-patients (accessed 29 December 2022).

NHS (2023) Healthy weight. Available at: www.nhs.uk/live-well/healthy-weight/bmi-calculator/ (accessed 24 July 2023).

NHS Digital (2022) Workforce statistics – July 2022. Available at: https://digital.nhs.uk/data-and-information/publications/statistical/nhs-workforce-statistics/july-2022 (accessed 22 March 2023).

NHS England (2018) Guidance for commissioners: interpreting and translation services in primary care. Available at: www.england.nhs.uk/wp-content/uploads/2018/09/guidance-for-commissioners-interpreting-and-translation-services-in-primary-care.pdf (accessed 5 March 2022).

NHS England (2020) Freedom to speak up – NHS improvement's raising concerns (whistleblowing) policy for NHS staff. Available at: www.england.nhs.uk/wp-content/uploads/2020/08/External_whistleblowing_policy_for_NHSI.pdf (accessed 7 November 2023).

NHS England (2021) Gender pay gap report. Available at: https://www.england.nhs.uk/wp-content/uploads/2021/10/B0986_iii_Gender-Pay-Gap-Report_2021.pdf (accessed 8 November 2022).

NHS England (2022) Understanding different types of bias. Available at: https://nshcs.hee.nhs.uk/about/equality-diversity-and-inclusion/conscious-inclusion/understanding-different-types-of-bias/ (accessed 1 November 2023).

NHS England (2023a) External freedom to speak up policy. Available at: www.england.nhs.uk/long-read/external-freedom-to-speak-up-policy-for-nhs-workers/ (accessed 14 November 2023).

NHS England (2023b) Patients to benefit from faster, more convenient care, under major new GP access recovery plan. Available at: www.england.nhs.uk/2023/05/patients-to-benefit-from-faster-more-convenient-care-under-major-new-gp-access-recovery-plan/ (accessed 1 November 2023).

NHS Providers (2020) BAME representation and experience in the NHS. Available at: https://nhsproviders.org/inclusive-leadership/bame-representation-and-experience-in-the-nhs (accessed 29 October 2022).

Noon, M (2018) Pointless diversity training: unconscious bias, new racism and agency work. *Employment and Society*, 32(1): 198–209.

Nursing and Midwifery Council (NMC) (2017) What sanctions are and when we might use them. Available at: www.nmc.org.uk/ftp-library/sanctions/the-sanctions/ (accessed 24 February 2023).

Nursing and Midwifery Council (NMC) (2018a) The Code. Available at: www.nmc.org.uk/globalassets/sitedocuments/nmc-publications/nmc-code.pdf (accessed 24 February 2023).

Nursing and Midwifery Council (NMC) (2018b) Standards of Proficiency for Nursing Associates. Available at: www.nmc.org.uk/globalassets/sitedocuments/education-standards/nursing-associates-proficiency-standards.pdf (accessed 24 February 2023).

Nursing and Midwifery Council (NMC) (2022a) Openness and honesty when things go wrong: the professional duty of candour. Available at: www.nmc.org.uk/globalassets/sitedocuments/nmc-publications/openness-and-honesty-professional-duty-of-candour.pdf (accessed 24 February 2023).

Nursing and Midwifery Council (NMC) (2022b) Corporate plan 2022–2025. Available at: www.nmc.org.uk/about-us/our-role/our-corporate-plan/ (accessed 24 February 2023).

Nursing and Midwifery Council (NMC) (2022c) Our Equality, Diversity, and Inclusion (EDI) Plan. Available at: www.nmc.org.uk/about-us/equality-diversity-and-inclusion/our-edi-aims/our-edi-plan/ (accessed 24 February 2023).

Nursing and Midwifery Council (NMC) (2022d) Professional indemnity arrangement. Available at: www.nmc.org.uk/registration/joining-the-register/professional-indemnity-arrangement (accessed 1 November 2023).

Nursing and Midwifery Council (NMC) (2023a) Registration data reports. Available at: www.nmc.org.uk/about-us/reports-and-accounts/registration-statistics/ (accessed 22 March 2023).

Nursing and Midwifery Council (2023b) An introduction to fitness to practise. Available at: www.nmc.org.uk/concerns-nurses-midwives/what-is-fitness-to-practise/an-introduction-to-fitness-to-practise/ (accessed 23 May 2023).

Nursing and Midwifery Council (NMC) (2023c) Our latest information about nursing and midwifery in the UK. Available at: www.nmc.org.uk/globalassets/sitedocuments/data-reports/may-2023/isl114-23-er-data-report_final_web-acc.pdf (accessed 16 August 2023).

Office of National Statistics (ONS) (2020) People population and community. Available at: www.ons.gov.uk/peoplepopulationandcommunity/birthsdeathsandmarriages/deaths/articles/deathsregisteredduetocovid19/2020 (accessed 29 December 2022).

Office National Statistics (ONS) (2022) Census 2021. Available at: www.ons.gov.uk/census/aboutcensus/legislationandpolicy (accessed 24 July 2023).

Orwell, G (1949) *Animal Farm*. London: Penguin Classics.

Parsons, T (1951) *The Social System*. Glencoe, IL: The Free Press.

Platt, E (2021) Why ethnic minorities are bearing the brunt of COVID-19. Available at: www.lse.ac.uk/research/research-for-the-world/race-equity/why-ethnic-minorities-are-bearing-the-brunt-of-covid-19 (accessed 29 December 2022).

Potter, L, Horwood, J, and Feder, G (2022) Access to healthcare for street sex workers in the UK: perspectives and best practice guidance from a national cross-sectional survey of frontline workers. *BMC Health Services Research*, 22: 179.

Public Health England (2016) Faith at end of life: a resource for professionals, providers and commissioners working in communities. Available at: www.gov.uk/government/publications/faith-at-end-of-life-public-health-approach-resource-for-professionals (accessed 7 November 2023).

Razaq, A, Harrison, D, Karunanithi, S, Barr, B, Asaria, M and Khunti, K (2020) BAME COVID-19 deaths – What do we know? Rapid Data and Evidence Review. The Centre for Evidence Based Medicine.

Roe v *Wade*, 410 U.S. 113 (1973).

Roper, N, Logan, W and Tierney, AJ (2000) *The Roper–Logan–Tierney Model of Nursing: Based on Activities of Living*. Harlow: Churchill Livingstone.

Shelter (2023) Legal definition of homelessness and threatened homelessness. Available at: https://england.shelter.org.uk/professional_resources/legal/homelessness_applications/homelessness_and_threatened_homelessness/legal_definition_of_homelessness_and_threatened_homelessness (accessed 1 November 2023).

Sickle Cell Society (2023) Available at: www.sicklecellsociety.org/about-sickle-cell/ (accessed 24 July 2023).

Sinnott-Armstrong, W (2022) 'Consequentialism', in Zalta, Edward N and Nodelman, Uri (eds) *The Stanford Encyclopedia of Philosophy* (Winter 2022 edn). Available online: https://plato.stanford.edu/archives/win2022/entries/consequentialism (accessed 1 November 2023).

Sippitt, A (2015) Job applicants with ethnic minority sounding names are less likely to be called for interview. London: Full Fact.

Social Care Institute for Excellence (SCIE) (2022) Deprivation of Liberty Safeguards (DoLS). Available at: www.scie.org.uk/mca/dols/at-a-glance (accessed 23 May 2023).

Staurowsky, EJ, Watanabe, N, Cooper, J, Cooky, C, Lough, N, Paule-Koba, A, Pharr, Williams, S, Cummings, S, Issokson-Silver, K and Snyder, M (2020) *Chasing Equity: The Triumphs, Challenges, and Opportunities in Sports for Girls and Women*. New York, NY: Women's Sports Foundation.

Stonewall (2017) LGBT in Britain – Trans Report. Available at: www.stonewall.org.uk/lgbt-britain-trans-report (accessed 29 December 2022).

Such, E, Jaipaul, R and Salway, S (2018) Modern slavery in the UK: how should the health sector be responding? *Journal of Public Health*, 42(1): 216–20.

Sulmasy, D (2007) 'Reinventing' the Rule of Double Effect, in Steinbock, Bonnie (ed) The Oxford Handbook of Bioethics. Oxford: Oxford University Press, pages 114–49.

Swihart, D, Yarrarapu, S and Martin, R (2022) *Cultural Religious Competence in Clinical Practice*. National Library of Medicine.

Thompson, N (2020) *Anti Discriminatory Practice* (7th edn). London: Red Globe Press.

Tsipursky, G and McRaney, D (2020) *The Blindspots Between Us: How to Overcome Unconscious Cognitive Bias and Build Better Relationships*. Oakland, CA: New Harbinger Publications.

West, SU (2019) Blog: Role differences between nursing associates and nurses. Available at: www.nmc.org.uk/news/news-and-updates/blog-whats-a-nursing-associate/ (accessed 1 November 2023).

White, A and Chanoff, D (2011) *Seeing Patients: Unconscious Bias in Health Care*. Harvard, MA: Harvard University Press.

World Health Organization (WHO) (2022) Abuse of older people. Available at: www.who.int/news-room/fact-sheets/detail/abuse-of-older-people (accessed 8 November 2022).

World Health Organization (WHO) (2023) Female genital mutilation. Available at: www.who.int/news-room/fact-sheets/detail/female-genital-mutilation#:~:text=Overview,organs%20for%20non%2Dmedical%20reasons (accessed 16 August 2023).

Wrottesley, SV, Prioreschi, A, Slemming, W, Cohen, E, Dennis, CL and Norris, SA (2020) Maternal perspectives on infant feeding practices in Soweto, South Africa. *Public Health Nutrition*, 24(12): 3602–14.

Index

Note: Page numbers in **bold** and *italics* represent tables and figures respectively.